# SEXUALLY AGGRESSIVE WOMEN

# SEXUALLY AGGRESSIVE WOMEN

## Current Perspectives and Controversies

Edited by
**PETER B. ANDERSON**
**CINDY STRUCKMAN-JOHNSON**

**THE GUILFORD PRESS**
New York    London

**Library of Congress Cataloging-in-Publication Data**

Sexually aggressive women: current perspectives and controversies/edited
by Peter B. Anderson, Cindy Struckman-Johnson.
    p.   cm.
    Includes bibliographical references and index.
    ISBN 1-57230-165-1
    1. Women—Sexual behavior. 2. Women—Psychology.
3. Aggressiveness (Psychology) I. Anderson, Peter B.
II. Struckman-Johnson, Cindy.
HQ29.S5 1998
306.7′082—dc21                         98-2635
                                       CIP

# Contributors

**Elizabeth Rice Allgeier** (PhD, Purdue University) is professor of psychology at Bowling Green State University, Ohio, where she was awarded the Alumni Association's Master Teacher Award in 1988 and was named Outstanding Contributor to Graduate Education in 1992. The author of numerous books, chapters, articles, and papers, she and her husband, Rick Allgeier, recently completed the fourth edition of *Sexual Interactions* (Heath, 1995). She was named the American Psychological Association's 1986 G. Stanley Hall Lecturer on Sexuality. Actively involved with the Society for the Scientific Study of Sexuality (SSSS), Allgeier has been an SSSS fellow since 1983 and served as its 1985–1986 president. She received the Kinsey Award for Outstanding Contributions to Sexual Science in 1994. Allgeier serves on the editorial boards of five journals and was editor of *The Journal of Sex Research* from 1993 to 1997.

**Peter B. Anderson**, PhD, is an associate professor of health and human sexuality education in the Department of Human Performance and Health Promotion at the University of New Orleans. Dr. Anderson received his doctorate from the human sexuality program of the Department of Health Education at New York University, where he had the opportunity to study in both Africa and Scandinavia. He and Deborah Richie, MA (Assistant Director of Housing for Academic Programs and Research, University of Illinois at Champaign–Urbana), later became leaders of the international study portion of NYU's program in human sexuality. This is Dr. Anderson's second edited volume. His first, *Does Anyone Still Remember When Sex Was Fun?: Positive Sexuality in the Age of AIDS* (Kendall/Hunt, 1990, 1992, 1994, 1996; with Diane deMauro and

v

Raymond J. Noonan), now in its third edition, continues to provide information and dialogue about HIV disease and AIDS. Dr. Anderson has worked, published, and studied in the area of human sexuality for the past 25 years.

**E. Sandra Byers, PhD,** is a professor of psychology at the University of New Brunswick in Fredericton, Canada. She also has a private practice in clinical psychology. She is the founding director of the Muriel McQueen Fergusson Centre for Family Violence Research at the University of New Brunswick. Dr. Byers has been working in the area of human sexuality for the past 20 years. She is the author or coauthor of more than 50 journal articles and book chapters and has recently coedited *Sexual Coercion in Dating Relationships* (Haworth, 1996), which also appeared as a special issue of *Journal of Psychology and Human Sexuality.* Dr. Byers is past president of the Canadian Sex Research Forum, is a fellow of the Society for the Scientific Study of Sexuality, a member of the advisory board of the Sex Information and Education Council of Council, and a consulting editor to the *Canadian Journal of Human Sexuality* and the *Journal of Psychology and Human Sexuality.*

**Lee Ellis** holds a PhD from Florida State University and has been teaching sociology and anthropology at Minot State University in Minot (rhymes with "why not"), North Dakota, since 1977. Dr. Ellis's primary interests include criminality, social stratification, and sex differences in behavior. Books written or edited by Dr. Ellis include *Theories of Rape* (Hemisphere, 1989), *Crime in Biological, Social, and Moral Contexts* (Praeger, 1990), *Social Stratification and Socioeconomic Inequality,* Volumes 1 and 2 (Praeger, 1993, 1994), *Sexual Orientation* (Praeger, 1997), and *Males, Females and Behavior: Toward Biological Understanding* (Praeger, 1998).

**Jennifer C. Lamping** (PhD, Bowling Green State University) is currently a faculty member at Sinclair College in Dayton, Ohio. While she was completing her graduate work at Bowling Green State University, she was awarded the 1995 Freeburne Graduate Student Teaching Award and served as the assistant editor of *The Journal of Sex Research* (1993–1994). Dr. Lamping has presented several papers at conferences based on her research on sexual coercion and other related topics. Her theoretical research on attributions about victims of mugging and rape was awarded Bowling Green State University's Sigma Xi Graduate Student Research Award in the psychology division in 1994.

**John G. Macchietto** served as a counseling psychologist and director of the Student Counseling Center at Tarleton State University in Stephenville, Texas, from 1984 to 1995. He is also a licensed professional counselor in Texas. Dr. Macchietto received his PhD in Counseling from the Counseling Psychology Department at the University of Kansas in

Lawrence, Kansas, in 1983. His work with men and men's issues is extensive. He worked from 1982 to 1984 in the Psychology Services of the Vietnam Post-traumatic Stress Unit of the Veterans Administration Medical Center in Topeka, Kansas. He also served on the board of directors of the National Coalition of Free Men for 7 years and served as the editor of *Transitions,* the national publication of this organization, for 3½ years. He has given several presentations on men's issues for communities, as well as professional organizations such as the American Counseling Association and the American Psychological Association. Presently, he is establishing himself in the music profession as a music publisher, composer, lyricist, producer, and performer.

**Charlene L. Muehlenhard** received her PhD in clinical psychology in 1981 from the University of Wisconsin, Madison. She is currently an associate professor at the University of Kansas, with a joint appointment in psychology and women's studies. Her research focuses on rape and other forms of sexual coercion, communication and miscommunication about sex, and other gender issues. She is a fellow of the American Psychological Association in Division 35, Psychology of Women, and was the 1996–1997 president of the Society for the Scientific Study of Sexuality (SSSS). She has been the director of the KU women's studies program, and is on the boards of directors of SSSS, the Douglas County Rape Victim/Survivor Service, and the Freedom Coalition, a group working for education and civil rights regarding LesBiGay issues.

**Lucia F. O'Sullivan,** received her PhD in social psychology under the supervision of Elizabeth Rice Allgeier from Bowling Green State University, Ohio, where she also served as assistant editor for *The Journal of Sex Research.* She is currently a postdoctorate research fellow at the HIV Center for Clinical and Behavioral Studies at Columbia University, New York. She was awarded a Sexuality Research Fellowship from the Social Science Research Council. This fellowship funded her 2-year study of the social cognitions of inner-city minority girls' sexual experiences. She has published a number of articles in the area of gender and sexuality and coedited *Sexual Coercion in Dating Relationships* (Haworth, 1996) with E. Sandra Byers.

**Andrea Parrot,** PhD, is a nationally recognized expert in the field of acquaintance rape and women's health and an associate professor at Cornell University, where she teaches up to 500 students per semester in a human sexuality course and in other courses related to health issues and medical ethics. She is also a clinical assistant professor of psychiatry at the State University of New York Health Sciences Center of Syracuse, New York. Dr. Parrot has published numerous books, manuscripts, and articles on the subject of acquaintance rape, including her most recent, *Rape*

*Prevention 101: Sexual Assault Education for Male College Athletes* (Learning Publications, 1994), and *Sexual Assault on Campus: The Problem and the Solution* (Lexington Books, 1993). Along with her scholarly work, Dr. Parrot is a consultant to many colleges, universities, federal and state agencies, and crime prevention and other agencies. She has been interviewed by many national magazines and on major radio and television talk shows such as *Good Morning America, Larry King Live, Face the Nation,* and *Oprah.*

**Mary E. Craig Shea** earned her doctorate in clinical psychology from the University of South Carolina in 1990. Her research has been primarily in areas of human sexuality, focusing on sexual coercion, assault, and abuse. She has published 15 articles and two book chapters and has presented more than 40 papers at national and regional conferences. Dr. Shea is currently employed as a medical and geriatric psychologist with the Department of Veterans Affairs and is in private practice in Columbia, South Carolina. She continues her academic and research involvement as an associate professor at the University of South Carolina School of Medicine.

**Wendy Stock** received her doctorate in clinical psychology from the State University of New York at Stony Brook in 1983. Her specialization areas are human sexuality, feminist issues in clinical psychology, and gender issues. Dr. Stock's research has focused on women's and men's responses to pornography and on women's experiences of pornography in their lives. Other publications have included feminist analyses of sexual dysfunction and sex therapy, power dynamics in relationships, and sexual coercion. Dr. Stock was invited to present her findings to the Attorney General's Commission on Pornography in 1985 and is currently conducting a community survey of women's experiences of pornography. After completing her doctorate, Dr. Stock spent 1 year as director of a sexual dysfunctions clinic in Florida. Subsequently, she served as a research scientist on an NIH grant at Texas A&M University, examining causes of male erectile dysfunction. In 1993, Dr. Stock returned to the Bay Area and is in full-time private practice.

**Cindy Struckman-Johnson** received her doctorate in social psychology from the University of Kentucky at Lexington. She is presently a professor of psychology the University of South Dakota, where she teaches courses in social psychology, sex roles, and sexuality. Dr. Struckman-Johnson is the recipient of numerous teaching awards and has gained special recognition for her course, "Understanding the Sexes." In collaboration with David Struckman-Johnson, she presently conducts research on sexual coercion of men in campus and prison settings, persuasive appeals for condom use, and seat-belt safety. Dr. Struckman-Johnson has served as a consulting editor for *The Journal of Sex Research*. In 1997, the Society for the Scientific Study of Sexuality awarded Cindy and David Struckman-Johnson the Beigel Award for research excellence for their work on sexual coercion of men and women in prison.

**David Struckman-Johnson** received his doctorate in psychology from the University of South Dakota. He currently holds a joint professorship in psychology and computer science at the University of South Dakota. He teaches courses in statistics, research methodology, evaluation research, human–computer interaction, and computer programming. His current research interests include sexual aggression, program evaluation in the area of child abuse and neglect, and traffic safety. Dr. Struckman-Johnson is currently a member of the technical team, under contract to the National Center on Child Abuse and Neglect, that is responsible for creation and analysis of the national child abuse and neglect database.

# Contents

   Coercion among College Women
   *Mary E. Craig Shea*

6. Why Some Sexual Assaults Are Not Committed             105
   by Men: A Biosocial Analysis
   *Lee Ellis*

              III. COMPARISONS OF MALE                    119
              AND FEMALE EXPERIENCES
              OF SEXUAL COERCION

7. The Dynamics and Impact of Sexual Coercion             121
   of Men by Women
   *Cindy Struckman-Johnson and David Struckman-Johnson*

8. Similar But Different: Men's and Women's               144
   Experiences of Sexual Coercion
   *E. Sandra Byers and Lucia F. O'Sullivan*

9. Women's Sexual Coercion of Men:                        169
   A Feminist Analysis
   *Wendy Stock*

           IV. TREATMENT AND PREVENTION                   185
              OF FEMALE SEXUAL AGGRESSION

10. Treatment Issues of Adult Male Victims                187
    of Female Sexual Aggression
    *John G. Macchietto*

11. Meaningful Sexual Assault Prevention Programs         205
    for Men
    *Andrea Parrot*

    Postscript: Where Do We Go from Here?                 225
    *Peter B. Anderson and Cindy Struckman-Johnson*

    Index                                                 237

# Introduction

PETER B. ANDERSON
CINDY STRUCKMAN-JOHNSON

We have created this edited volume to challenge prevailing assumptions about the nature of sexual relations between adult heterosexual women and men. We propose that, contrary to stereotypes that women are sexually passive and "uninterested," there are women who demand, pressure, extort, and even force adult and adolescent men into sexual interactions. In the chapters that follow, contributing authors explore questions about the conceptual issues related to the study of sexually aggressive women, the characteristics and motives of women who use sexual aggression, the nature of men's reactions to female sexual aggression, and new directions in research, prevention, and therapy.

In publishing this volume, our primary goal is to bring attention to the small but significant body of research on sexually aggressive women and the men they pursue. Our other purpose is to air the myriad controversies surrounding this research. Currently, there are arguments about definitions of sexual aggression, appropriateness of research design and methods, subjectivity and bias in measures, and the political implications of the results. One of the greatest points of conflict is whether or not this research detracts from the literature on sexual coercion of women by men.

Our own experiences as researchers in academe have underscored the need for this book. Peter Anderson, upon entering the PhD program in human sexuality at New York University in 1986, received a recommendation from a friend to investigate the topic of women who rape men. Upon reviewing the literature, Peter found this area to be virtually unstudied. Only one classic study on sexual molestation of men by women (Sarrel & Masters, 1982) was available. Realizing that research in this area would substantially advance knowledge in the field, Peter chose the dissertation topic of women's sexual aggression toward adolescent and adult men. Peter quickly discovered that his choice was controversial. Some colleagues told him his research was potentially damaging to women's causes. Others warned him that his work would never be published because of the attitudes of some people sitting on editorial review boards. Contrary to prediction, Peter published various findings from his dissertation research in the *Archives of Sexual Behavior* (Anderson & Aymami, 1993) and *Sexual Abuse: A Journal of Research and Treatment* (Anderson, 1996).

Cindy Struckman-Johnson, professor of psychology at the University of South Dakota, also encountered interesting reactions to her research. In 1985, she distributed a survey about sexuality and birth control to more than 600 students on campus. Because of national publicity about date rape, she included one question about forced sex on dates. As expected, 22% of the women said that they had experienced at least one incident of forced sexual intercourse in high school or college dating. To her amazement, 16% of the men reported the same experience! Mystified by the outcome, Cindy administered a follow-up survey to half of her participants to obtain more information from victims. Ultimately, she obtained data from 22 men who described how they were forced to have sex with dates by emotional demands, blackmail, intoxication, and some use of physical restraint.

After Cindy presented these results at a conference in Chicago (Struckman-Johnson, 1986), the media reacted to the findings with amusement and disbelief. Dozens of newspapers throughout the country carried the article with lighthearted bylines such as "Coeds Turn Tables on Men," "Predator Females Found in South Dakota," and "It Wasn't Like This When I Went to School." *Playboy* magazine featured the story in its "Forum," accompanied by a cartoon of a woman capturing a fleeing man with a giant net ("Date Rape," 1987).

The responses of professionals in academe were mixed. Some of Cindy's colleagues told others that men had most likely given false reports on the survey. Several well-known researchers in the area commented that the reporting of men's somewhat "harmless" experiences of forced sex trivialized the real problem of rape of women. However, the paper received favorable attention from Dr. Elizabeth Rice Allgeier, then associate editor of *The Journal of Sex Research,* and it was published in 1988 (Struckman-Johnson, 1988).

In retrospect, we are not surprised by the reactions to our research. In the 1970s and 1980s, the literature on sexual norms indicated that women's role is to regulate and restrict men's sexual advances, whereas men's role is to initiate and press for sex at every opportunity (e.g., Clark & Hatfield, 1989; McCormick, Brannigan, & LaPlant, 1984; Simon & Gagnon, 1986). In dramatic contrast, our findings suggested that many women are clearly interested in sex and will overtly and sometimes aggressively initiate sexual activity. Men, contrary to stereotypes, are not interested in every sexual opportunity but usually restrict their sexual activity for appropriate partners and situations.

By the late 1980s, a trickle of studies supported this new perspective on male–female sexual relations. The most influential of these was a study by Muehlenhard and Cook (1988) that revealed that substantial percentages of women and men at Texas A&M University had engaged in unwanted sexual activity at some time in their lives. Results of this now-famous work were widely cited in the academic and popular literature and stirred interest in the topic of sexually aggressive women.

However, change was slow to come. By the early 1990s, the great majority of published studies on sexual coercion still exclusively conceptualized women as passive victims and men as sexual predators. Thus, we welcomed a proposal by The Guilford Press to publish research on sexually aggressive women. Our first task was to extend an open invitation to numerous researchers in sexual coercion to contribute chapters to the book. Ultimately, 13 researchers from the United States and Canada have contributed chapters on their research.

We have organized the contributors' chapters into four sections.

The volume begins with perspectives on dilemmas associated with the methods and politics of conducting research on sexually aggressive women. In Section II, research on the characteristics and motives of sexually aggressive woman is presented. Section III is devoted to comparisons of the male and female experiences of sexual victimization, and the final section focuses on treatment and prevention issues.

There are several features of the book that require clarification. First, this book is not exclusively about women who use physical force to obtain sex. We define female heterosexual aggression as an act in which a woman uses pressure or force to obtain sexual contact with an adolescent or adult man against his will. Our contributing authors have documented that only small percentages of women use force tactics such as physical restraint, the threat or use of physical harm, or the use of weapons. For the most part, our contributors are writing about women who have used pressure tactics such as verbal demands, emotional manipulation, deception, blackmail, and intoxication to gain sexual access to reluctant men.

Although we do not intend to discriminate, this book is about sexual interactions between *heterosexual* women and men. Sexual aggression in lesbian and gay relationships, or perpetrated against men by men who define themselves as heterosexual, are also critical areas of research, but they are beyond the scope of this volume. In addition, this volume focuses on *adult* women and their interactions with *adult* and *adolescent* men. Although there is literature on women of all ages being sexually aggressive toward children, we chose to limit our topic to adult women's sexual aggression toward adolescent or adult men.

Given the preliminary state of research and theory on this topic, this book cannot provide a definitive answer to why women engage in sexual aggression. However, our volume does represent a major first step toward this purpose. We have brought together the groundbreaking work of many of the first researchers to study female sexual aggression. Each of our contributing authors presents a unique analysis and perspective on women's heterosexual aggression. It is our hope that the rich variety of ideas and findings of our contributors will stimulate research to further develop this field.

Finally, this volume is not intended to encourage people to take "sides" on issues about sexually aggressive women. Scientific explanations of the problem of sexual aggression between the sexes will not be advanced as long as people are polarized by seemingly opposite viewpoints. For example, there is a great temptation to view research on aggressive females and male victims as "pro-men" and research on male aggressors and female victims as "pro-women." There have been acrimonious divisions between those who believe that sexual coercion is motivated by power and anger and those who propose that sexual interest may be a causal factor. Feminist and culturally based perspectives on sexual coercion have been pitted against evolutionary and biologically based theories (Muehlenhard, Harney, & Jones, 1992). We agree with Hare-Mustin and Marecek (1990), who wrote: "In western society, we easily slide into a focus on differences and dualities when we organize the world about us. Psychology is part of this tradition based on operations of comparing and contrasting. But to see both sides of a problem is the surest way to prevent its solution because there are always more than two sides" (p. 1).

Thus, we offer in this volume a variety of viewpoints to illuminate the complexity of this subject. An array of theoretical perspectives is represented, including social learning, feminist, biosocial, and evolutionary theories. We anticipate that our readers will find points of common ground, all of which may foster greater understanding of the nature of sexual relations between women and men.

## REFERENCES

Anderson, P. B. (1996). Correlates of college women's self-reports of heterosexual aggression. *Sexual Abuse: A Journal of Research and Treatment, 8*(2), 121–131.

Anderson, P. B., & Aymami, R. (1993). Reports of female initiation of sexual contact: Male and female differences. *Archives of Sexual Behavior, 22*(4), 335–343.

Clark, R., & Hatfield, E. (1989). Gender differences in receptivity to sexual offers. *Journal of Psychology and Human Sexuality, 2,* 39–55.

Date rape. (1987, February). *Playboy, 34,* 47.

Hare-Mustin, R., & Marecek, J. (Eds.). (1990). *Making a difference: Psychology and the construction of gender.* New Haven, CT: Yale University Press.

McCormick, N., Brannigan, G., & LaPlant, M. (1984). Social desirability in the bedroom: Role of approval motivation in sexual relationships. *Sex Roles, 11,* 303–314.

Muehlenhard, C., & Cook, S. (1988). Men's self-reports of unwanted sexual activity. *Journal of Sex Research, 24,* 58–72.

Muehlenhard, C., Harney, P., & Jones, J. (1992). From "victim precipitated rape" to "date rape": How far have we come? *Annual Review of Sex Research, 3,* 219–252.

Sarrel, P., & Masters, W. (1982). Sexual molestation of men by women. *Archives of Sexual Behavior, 11,* 117–131.

Simon, W., & Gagnon, J. (1986). Sexual scripts: Permanence and change. *Archives of Sexual Behavior, 15,* 97–120.

Struckman-Johnson, C. (1986, May). *Forced sex on dates: It happens to men, too.* Paper presented at the annual meeting of the Midwestern Psychological Association, Chicago.

Struckman-Johnson, C. (1988). Forced sex on dates: It happens to men, too. *Journal of Sex Research, 24,* 234–241.

# I

---

# RESEARCH AND
# CONCEPTUAL ISSUES
# IN STUDYING SEXUALLY
# AGGRESSIVE WOMEN

In our first section, we take the liberty as coeditors of expressing our concerns about barriers to conducting research on sexually aggressive women and their male targets. Extending this theme, Charlene L. Muehlenhard in Chapter 2 frames the debate for the question, Should we study the sexually aggressive woman? Muehlenhard is one of the nation's top researchers and philosophers in the sexual coercion area. She is ideally suited to write this chapter, as she has conducted significant research on sexual coercion of women by men yet was one of the first to document men's reports of engaging in unwanted sexual activity. Muehlenhard sets the stage by discussing the concept of gender and the polarizing issue of whether women and men are perceived to be similar or different. She then invites the reader to weigh the benefits of new knowledge and theories gained from studying female sexual aggression against potential costs to the status and welfare of women.

In Chapter 3, Elizabeth Rice Allgeier and Jennifer C. Lamping address the politics of research on sexual coercion. Allgeier, past editor of the highly esteemed *Journal of Sex Research,* and Lamping suggest that one's theoretical and political views about sexual coercion may inherently bias his or her research questions, choices for design and measures, and interpretation of results. They expose the "midpoint problem" that has resulted in misleading interpretations of scalar ratings in well-known studies. Their most startling revelation is that a measure used in hundreds of sexual coercion surveys does not accurately assess behaviors. We anticipate that this chapter will be recommended reading for present and future researchers in the sexual coercion area.

# 1

# "Men Do and Women Don't": Difficulties in Researching Sexually Aggressive Women

CINDY STRUCKMAN-JOHNSON
PETER B. ANDERSON

Why are there so few studies on sexually aggressive women and why are the results of this research often discounted? In this chapter, we review three factors that have hindered this field of study: (1) acceptance of the myth that women can do no harm; (2) the failure of investigators to ask women and men about female sexual aggression; and (3) existence of a double standard in defining male and female sexual aggression. We also offer remedies for aspects of the problems.

## THE MYTH THAT WOMEN CAN DO NO HARM

One of the most perplexing research problems we have encountered is public and professional skepticism about the concept of sexually

9

aggressive women. Essentially, people tell us that "women don't do this sort of thing," and if they did, "wouldn't men be lucky!" Consequently, there is little research interest in a behavior considered so rare or atypical. This skepticism reflects a prevailing view that the female human is largely incapable of causing physical harm to other persons—children or adults. Meta-analyses of research on physical aggression confirm that, compared to men, women do engage in less physically harmful behavior in experimental settings, although there are some situations in which men and women behave similarly (e.g., Bettencourt & Miller, 1996; Eagly & Steffen, 1986). However, research has also revealed that there are real-life circumstances in which some women do inflict physical harm. For example, Straus (1993) discovered in numerous national surveys that men and women had similar rates of violent behavior toward their spouses, although women were more likely to be injured in incidents. Although most women reported acting in self-defense, in nearly half of the cases women reported initiating the aggression. In one-fourth of the households, the woman was the sole abuser. In a study of interpersonal violence among college students, Lottes and Weinberg (1996) found that higher percentages of women than men reported slapping, biting, and kicking their dating partners. Mould (1990) and Fillion (1996) have argued that the statistics on female abuse of male partners have been ignored or suppressed in the literature because they belie the prevalent feminist portrayal of men as predators and women as victims.

Another discomfiting image is that of women as child sexual abusers. Although most perpetrators of child sexual abuse are men, numerous studies have found that a substantial portion of abusers are girls or women. For example, in a study by Fritz, Stoll, and Wagner (1981), 60% of male victims of child sexual abuse reported being victimized by women. Other studies have established that 16% (Finkelhor, 1979), 27% (Gebhard, Gagnon, Pomeroy, & Christenson, 1965), and 14% (Bell & Weinberg, 1981) of male victims had been sexually abused by women acting either alone or with a partner. In their landmark study, *The Social Organization of Sexuality,* Laumann, Gagnon, Michael, and Michaels (1994) reported that 7% of male respondents had had childhood sexual contact with an older girl or woman. Confronting the mentality that "Men do and women don't," Allen (1991) has noted that professionals have traditionally resisted information about women who sexually abuse their own and other children.

The myth that women do not sexually aggress against adult men is supported by numerous stereotypes and misconceptions. One influential stereotype is that women's role is to restrict and to control sexual activity in dating relationships, whereas men's role is to initiate sex (e.g., Clark & Hatfield, 1989). Therefore, some people do not think that women—especially "nice" women—would ask their dating partner for sex, let alone exert pressure or force to obtain it. However, research by our contributing authors E. Sandra Byers and Lucia O'Sullivan (Chapter 8) and Peter B. Anderson (Chapter 4) reveals that the traditional dating script is eroding and that women now commonly initiate sexual activity using both positive and negative strategies. A related stereotype is that women have low sex drives (e.g., Chalker, 1994) and therefore do not have sufficient desire to force a man into sex. In Chapter 6, contributing author Lee Ellis suggests that, in accordance with his biosocial theory, a small percentage of women may be motivated by a strong sex drive and other related qualities to commit sexual assault.

Another belief is that the average woman does not have the size, strength, or ability to physically force a man to have sexual contact (Struckman-Johnson & Struckman-Johnson, 1992). For example, contributing author Wendy Stock notes in Chapter 9 that men typically have the option of escaping or walking away from a sexually coercive woman. Nonetheless, researchers have discovered that women can accomplish forceful sexual aggression of men by using intimidation tactics, the assistance of other persons, and weapons. For example, Sarrel and Masters (1982) described an incident where a young man was tied up and forced to engage in sex with a woman who threatened him with a scalpel. Struckman-Johnson and Struckman-Johnson (1994) and others (e.g., Muehlen-hard & Cook, 1988) have also documented that many men reported engaging in unwanted sexual encounters because they were too intoxicated to give consent or to fend off a woman. As revealed by Cindy and David Struckman-Johnson in Chapter 7, alcohol is the "great leveler" of men's physical abilities to avoid coercive sexual contact with women.

Finally, there is the belief that it is impossible for a woman to have sexual relations with a man who does not desire her (Sarrel & Masters, 1982). The specific question is, How can a woman accomplish penile–vaginal intercourse with a reluctant man with a limp penis? Sarrel and Masters (1982) explained that men can experience sexual arousal due to touch stimulation or strong emotional reactions, such as fear, even when they do not have any psychological desire for a female initiator. They cited an example in which a group of women tied a man to a bed and mounted him repeatedly for sexual intercourse. The women used manual stimulation and a knife pressed against his scrotum to force the man to have erections. In Chapter 7, Cindy and David Struckman-Johnson's research reveals that women can be quite adept at finding ways to mount the erect penis of nonconsenting and/or intoxicated men. According to the Struckman-Johnsons, people tend to assume that female sexual aggression only involves penile–vaginal intercourse and overlook the more "manageable" acts of manual and oral stimulation of the penis. In their research, men commonly report that women engage in nonconsensual "penis grabbing" and fellatio.

## NEGLECTING TO ASSESS FEMALE SEXUAL AGGRESSION

Further limiting our knowledge of this subject, many researchers fail to ask questions about female sexual aggression. Perhaps because of assumptions that women do not engage in sexual aggression, researchers have routinely asked women *only* about victimization and men *only* about perpetration experiences. This outcome is encouraged by the use of instruments such as the Sexual Experiences Survey (SES; Koss & Oros, 1982), in which women answer questions about receiving sexual aggression and men respond to parallel questions about perpetrating the behavior. Another problem—rare to our knowledge—is the practice of collecting data on both female and male victimization but reporting only the results for female victimization (e.g., Sandberg, Jackson, & Petretic-Jackson, 1985).

Some researchers ask women and men about receiving and perpetrating sexual aggression but do so in a way that still emphasizes the incidence of female victimization. For example, in an important study of sexual aggression in the United States and Sweden, Lottes and Weinberg (1996) queried both women and men about receiving and perpetrating *nonphysical* sexual aggression. However, for acts of *physical* sexual aggression, only women were asked about victimization and only men were asked about perpetration. Consequently, women, but not men, were described as victims of serious levels of sexual aggression.

Another example is the *Social Organization of Sexuality* study (Laumann et al., 1994), which reported that 21.6% of the women and 1.5% of the men had been forced into sexual activity by an opposite-gender person. However, the authors explained that the 22% figure reflected women's responses to a confidential survey question that read, "Have you ever been forced by a man to do something that you did not want to?" The item was supposed to read "something *sexual*" but was misprinted. In a footnote, they add that 15% of women answered yes when the question was phrased correctly in the face-to-face interview (pp. 333–335). Fillion (1996) noted that what the authors call a "union" of women's responses is actually the higher rate obtained from the misprinted question.

Regarding the percentage of men sexually forced by women, Laumann et al. (1994) explained that the 1.5% rate was derived only from the face-to-face interview question (a situation where men may be reluctant to admit victimization). The authors *neglected to ask* men in the confidential survey if a woman had ever forced them to do something sexual. Laumann et al. cautioned that their measures of forced sex were broad in scope (i.e., the items referred to any type of sexual act) and "suspect" due to the misprint. Nonetheless, their estimates are now widely cited in the literature by those who may be unaware of the significant qualifications.

These assessment biases most likely reflect researchers' good intentions to draw attention to the important social problem of female sexual victimization. Undoubtedly, most researchers in the sexual-aggression area, including ourselves, desire to present our data in ways that convince the scientific world and the public that problems exist, merit further study, and require solutions. We must take care that our efforts do not inadvertently obscure or exaggerate the dimensions of the problem.

## DOUBLE STANDARDS FOR DEFINING SEXUAL AGGRESSION

We propose that a double standard of sexual aggression causes people to excuse acts of female sexual aggression reported in current research. There have long been "separate and unequal" standards for defining sexually coercive acts of women and men. From the 1950s through the 1970s, any sexual advances by women were considered to be "improper," "unladylike," and "aggressive" (Henley & Freeman, 1984). Thus, a college-age woman could have been labeled "sexually aggressive" if she asked a new dating partner to engage in sex, even though her behavior involved no pressure or force.

By comparison, standards defining inappropriate sexual initiatives of men were quite lenient. A college-age man's offer to engage in sex with a new dating partner would have been considered an expected or normal sexual initiative. According to studies of dating practices in these decades, men who did use forceful sexual initiatives may not have been labeled sexually aggressive. Kirkpatrick and Kanin (1957) found that nearly half of college women surveyed had experienced "offensive" or "displeasing" attempts by men to have sex. This estimate was replicated by Kanin and Parcell (1977), who observed that male sexual aggression was "normative," even when it escalated to forceful acts. A major survey of attitudes about sex and dating conducted in the 1970s indicated that many adolescent boys and girls judged it acceptable for a man to use force to have sex with a woman in some dating circumstances—such as when "she gets him sexually excited" (Goodchilds, Zellman, Johnson, & Giarrusso, 1988). In fact, there was not even a term to characterize this type of male sexual aggression until the 1980s, when the phrase "date rape" was coined (Bechhofer & Parrot, 1991).

From the 1980s until the present, there has been a reversal in these standards. Due to intense research and growing public awareness of the scope of sexual assault, men's sexual initiatives are now held to stricter standards of acceptability. Definitions of male sexual aggression now include pressure tactics such as continual arguments, deception, and use of authority, as well as force tactics of intimidation, physical restraint, harm, threats of harm, and use of alcohol and drugs to diminish one's ability to consent (e.g., Koss & Oros, 1982).

In contrast, we contend that the use of pressure tactics and even the use of some force tactics may be considered acceptable for today's sexually active woman. Many studies have shown that there is more social support for women who violate minor sexual norms, such as in "stealing a kiss," than there is for men who commit the identical action (e.g., Margolin, 1990; Semonsky & Rosenfeld, 1994).

Struckman-Johnson and Struckman-Johnson (1991) discovered that both men and women judged a range of coercive sexual strategies (e.g., verbal pressure, persistent stimulation, mock force, intoxication, and physical force) as unacceptable. However, male participants rated all acts as significantly more acceptable when the woman perpetrated them against a man as compared to when a man perpetrated them against a woman. Results of these studies suggest that sexual violations by a woman are seen as romantic and motivated by intimacy, whereas the identical behaviors by men are viewed as threatening, aggressive, and motivated by power and control.

We have found a similar tendency to redefine female sexual aggression as "romance" when we present our findings in public and professional forums. To paraphrase the actual reactions of some people in our audiences, a woman who persistently demands sex from a reluctant man is viewed as "expressing her sexuality"; a woman who persistently kisses, touches, and removes clothing from a reluctant man is being "seductive"; a woman who uses physical restraint to sit on a man or lock him in a room is being "playful"; and a woman who initiates sex with a drunken man is "way too horny for her own good." Some of these same actions by a man could potentially result in criminal prosecution.

We speculate that the more lenient standard for women is partly based on the belief that women would not really harm anyone. It may also reflect the new sexual norm that emphasizes the importance of women's sexual fulfillment and expects women to be active in that process (O'Sullivan & Byers, 1993). Whatever the source of the double standard, we believe that it fosters the perception that the study of female sexual aggression is about minor violations of sexual conduct.

## REMEDIES

We have several suggestions for ameliorating problems in research on female sexual aggression. It is important that researchers recognize that women *can* do harm to others in their quest for sexual intimacy and that men, despite assumptions about their physical and emotional invulnerability to female sexual aggression, *can* fall prey to pressure and force tactics used by a woman.

Our recommendation for the "failure to assess" problem is

straightforward: Social scientists who are undertaking surveys of the general prevalence of sexual aggression should include measures for victimization and perpetration for *both* male and female respondents. When presenting and discussing their findings, researchers should not focus exclusively on female sexual victimization but should provide a balance of information on female and male perpetration and male victimization.

The double standard for male and female aggression is most difficult to remedy. In fact, this dilemma is debated in several chapters of this volume. The egalitarian argument is that, in fairness, women and men should be held to the same standards of appropriate sexual conduct. However, another position (see Charlene L. Muehlenhard, Chapter 2; E. Sandra Byers & Lucia F. O'Sullivan, Chapter 8; and Wendy Stock, Chapter 9) argues that the motives, tactics, capacity to harm, and the impact of sexual aggression committed by women may intrinsically differ from the actions committed by men. Therefore, *separate* standards defining sexual aggression for the sexes may be appropriate.

Whether a single or dual standard is the ultimate outcome, we recommend that objectivity be applied to the analysis of behavior of both women and men. Perhaps our most important recommendation is to encourage social scientists to keep an open mind about the behaviors of women and men in sexually coercive interactions.

## REFERENCES

Allen, C. (1991). *Women and men as sexual abusers of children: A comparative analysis.* Orwell, VT: Safer Society Press.

Bechhofer, L., & Parrot, A. (1991). What is acquaintance rape? In A. Parrot & L. Bechhofer (Eds.), *Acquaintance rape: The hidden crime* (pp. 9–25). New York: Wiley.

Bell, A., & Weinberg, M. (1981). *Sexual preference: Its development among men and women.* Bloomington, IN: Indiana University Press.

Bettencourt, B., & Miller, N. (1996). Sex differences in aggression as a function of provocation: A meta-analysis. *Psychological Bulletin, 119,* 422–447.

Chalker, R. (1994). Updating the model of female sexuality. *SIECUS Report, 22,* 1–6.

Clark, R. D., & Hatfield, E. (1989). Gender differences in receptivity to sexual offers. *Journal of Psychology and Human Sexuality, 2,* 39–55.

Eagly, A. H., & Steffen, V. (1986). Gender and aggressive behavior: A meta-analytic review of the social psychological literature. *Psychological Bulletin, 100,* 309–330.

Fillion, K. (1996). Lip service: The truth about women's darker side in love, sex and friendship. New York: HarperCollins.

Finkelhor, D. (1979). *Sexually victimized children.* New York: Free Press.

Fritz, G., Stoll, K., & Wagner, N. (1981). A comparison of males and females who were sexually molested as children. *Journal of Sex and Marital Therapy, 7,* 54–58.

Gebhard, P. H., Gagnon, J. H., Pomeroy, W. B., & Christenson, C. V. (1965). *Sex offenders: An analysis of types.* New York: Harper & Row.

Goodchilds, J. D., Zellman, G. L., Johnson, P. B., & Giarrusso, R. (1988). Adolescents and their perceptions of sexual interactions. In A. W. Burgess (Ed.), *Rape and sexual assault II* (pp. 245–270). New York: Garland.

Henley, M., & Freeman, J. (1984). The sexual politics of interpersonal behavior. In J. Freeman (Ed.), *Women: A feminist perspective* (pp. 457–469). Mountain View, CA: Mayfield.

Kanin, E. J., & Parcell, S. R. (1977). Sexual aggression: A second look at the offended female. *Archives of Sexual Behavior, 6,* 67–76.

Kirkpatrick, C., & Kanin, E. (1957). Male sex aggression on a university campus. *American Sociological Review, 22,* 52–58.

Koss, M. P., & Oros, C. J. (1982). Sexual Experiences Survey: A research instrument investigating sexual aggression and victimization. *Journal of Consulting and Clinical Psychology, 50,* 455–457.

Laumann, E. O., Gagnon, J. H., Michael, R. T., & Michaels, S. (1994). *The social organization of sexuality: Sexual practices in the United States.* Chicago: University of Chicago Press.

Lottes, I., & Weinberg, M. (1996). Sexual coercion among university students: A comparison of the United States and Sweden. *Journal of Sex Research, 34,* 67–76.

Margolin, L. (1990). Gender and the stolen kiss: The social support of males and females to violate a partner's sexual consent in a noncoercive situation. *Archives of Sexual Behavior, 19,* 281–291.

Mould, D. (1990). Data base or data bias? *American Psychologist, 45,* 677.

Muehlenhard, C., & Cook, S. (1988). Men's self-reports of unwanted sexual activity. *Journal of Sex Research, 24,* 58–72.

O'Sullivan, L. F., & Byers, E. S. (1993). Eroding stereotypes: College women's attempts to influence reluctant male sexual partners. *Journal of Sex Research, 30,* 270–282.

Sandberg, G. G., Jackson, T. L., & Petretic-Jackson, P. J. (1985, May). *Sexual aggression and courtship violence in dating relationships.* Paper presented at the annual meeting of the Midwestern Psychological Association, Chicago.

Sarrel, P. M., & Masters, W. H. (1982). Sexual molestation of men by women. *Archives of Sexual Behavior, 11,* 117–131.

Semonsky, M. R., & Rosenfeld, L. B. (1994). Perceptions of sexual violations: Denying a kiss, stealing a kiss. *Sex Roles, 30,* 503–520.

Straus, M. A. (1993). Physical assaults by wives: A major social problem. In R. J. Gelles & D. R. Loseke (Eds.), *Current controversies on family violence* (pp. 67–87). Newbury Park, CA: Sage.

Struckman-Johnson, C. J., & Struckman-Johnson, D. L. (1991). Men's and women's acceptance of coercive sexual strategies varied by initiator gender and couple intimacy. *Sex Roles, 25,* 661–676.

Struckman-Johnson, C. J., & Struckman-Johnson, D. L. (1992). Acceptance of male rape myths among college men and women. *Sex Roles, 27,* 85–100.

Struckman-Johnson, C. J., & Struckman-Johnson, D. L. (1994). Men pressured and forced into sexual experience. *Archives of Sexual Behavior, 23,* 93–114.

# 2

# The Importance and Danger of Studying Sexually Aggressive Women

CHARLENE L. MUEHLENHARD

While having dinner at a meeting of the American Psychological Association, I got into a discussion with a fellow rape researcher. We argued about the role of gender in research on sexual coercion. Both of us had done studies investigating women's experiences as victims and men's experiences as perpetrators. When doing these studies, I had noticed that occasionally a male research participant would write in the questionnaire margins that he had been sexually coerced by a woman. After reading a few of these unsolicited comments, I had decided to study unwanted sexual activity experienced by men. One of my students and I then conducted a study in which we asked both women and men identical questions about their experiences with unwanted sexual activity (Muehlenhard & Cook, 1988). We found—to our surprise—that more men than women reported having engaged in unwanted sexual intercourse. Most often the unwanted intercourse that men reported was due to peer pressure and the pressures of adhering to gender stereotypes, but sometimes it was due to verbal or even physical pressure from their partners.

During our dinner conversation, my colleague argued that researchers should not ask women and men identical questions about sexual coercion because women and men have different experiences. I replied that we should ask women and men identical questions because, until we do, we will not know how different their experiences really are. She claimed that research on female perpetrators or male victims could be used against women; I argued that for too long scientists' uncritical acceptance of gender stereotypes has hurt women and that we should not perpetuate such stereotypes. She argued that even if women and men answered questions the same way, their experiences would have different meanings. I argued that this is an empirical question—that to learn about what sexual coercion means to both women and men, we need to ask them.

Who was right?

In this chapter, I explore the importance—but also the danger—of studying sexually aggressive women. There are many arguments for why we should study sexually aggressive women but also many reasons why this could be a dangerous endeavor. Before addressing these arguments specifically, however, I have included a section on the nature of gender. I included this section because gender is crucial to the controversy over studying sexually aggressive women. That is, this controversy is not about the value of *studying* important social problems, nor is it about whether *sexual aggression* is an important topic that deserves study. The controversy is not about studying sexually aggressive *men*; it is about studying sexually aggressive *women*. Hence, the nature of the distinctions between men and women and the meaning of gender are at the heart of this discussion. Thus, I devote the next several pages to a discussion of background issues and key concepts related to gender that provide the groundwork for the rest of the chapter. Using these concepts, I then turn to both the importance and the danger of studying sexually aggressive women.

## THE CONCEPT OF GENDER

Viewed one way, everyone knows what gender is, what a woman is, what a man is. Viewed another way, however, there are many different theories of gender, including both informal theories constructed by the general public and formal theories constructed by scholars. Different theories have different emphases. Some theories emphasize gender *differences*; others emphasize gender *similarities*; still others go beyond the difference–similarity question.

## Theories Focusing on Gender Differences

Focusing on gender differences is certainly popular in this culture. Examples are numerous: According to the traditional rhyme, girls are made of "sugar and spice and everything nice"; boys are made of "snips and snails and puppy dog tails." According to the recent pop psychology best-seller, "men are from Mars; women are from Venus" (Gray, 1994). And so on.

McFadden (1984) referred to theorists who emphasize gender differences as *maximizers*. Hare-Mustin and Marecek (1990) referred to "the view of male and female as different and opposite and thus as having mutually exclusive qualities" (pp. 30–31) as *alpha bias*. They took this term from the statistical concept of alpha, or Type I, errors, in which researchers conclude that there are group differences when in fact there are not.

Focusing on gender differences does not necessitate any one political stance (McFadden, 1984). Maximizers can range from conservative (i.e., aiming to preserve the status quo) to radical (i.e., aiming to transform the status quo; McFadden, 1984). At the conservative end of this continuum are traditional stereotyped views in which men are logical and strong and women are emotional and weak, in which men move in the public sphere and women are restricted to the private sphere, and in which characteristics ascribed to men are valued more than characteristics ascribed to women (this view is exemplified in popular writings such as those of Andelin, 1980, and Broverman, Vogel, Broverman, Clarkson, & Rosenkrantz, 1972, who documented similar views among college students and mental health professionals). A feminist concept of gender that focuses on differences is one that asserts that there are gender differences but celebrates these differences, valuing the characteristics ascribed to women as much as or more than the characteristics ascribed to men (e.g., Gilligan's [1982] view that women speak in a different moral voice than do men, and ecofeminists' views of women as more connected to nature than are men; Alaimo, 1994). At the most radical end of the continuum are feminist and lesbian separatists, who advocate that women can only be free when separated from men, either with separate institutions or with geographically separate space (e.g., Hoagland & Penelope, 1988).

## A Critique of Gender-Differences Approaches

Until recently, social scientists have approached the study of gender primarily through differences (Deaux & Major, 1990; Hare-Mustin & Marecek, 1990). This focus has in many ways led to exaggerated notions of gender differences. For example, studies finding no gender differences are often considered failures; studies are more likely to be published when results reveal gender differences than when they reveal no gender differences (Unger & Crawford, 1992). Statistically significant gender differences are emphasized and publicized by the mass media even when these differences are so small that they are of no practical significance (Hare-Mustin & Marecek, 1990; Unger & Crawford, 1992). Even when a gender difference is considered "moderate" or "large," the data almost always reveal considerable variation within each gender and considerable overlap between the genders; nevertheless, these results are often summarized as dichotomies or opposites, such as "men are aggressive; women are not aggressive" (Hare-Mustin & Marecek, 1990; Tavris, 1992; Unger & Crawford, 1992). Thus, in many ways, focusing on gender differences "obscures the commonalities between women and men" (Hare-Mustin & Marecek, 1990, p. 17), even discouraging the examination of such similarities (Unger, 1990). This approach leads to exaggerated, unrealistic impressions of women and men as opposites.

Empirical examination of popularly accepted gender differences has revealed most of them to be "either nonexistent, relatively insubstantial, or erratic in their patterns" (Morawski, 1987, p. 46). Some supposed gender differences have not been empirically supported (e.g., supposed gender differences in moral reasoning; see Colby & Damon, 1987). Others have been shown to be confounded with power (e.g., "men's" speech patterns turn out to be those used by people with power, regardless of their gender; "women's" speech patterns turn out to be those used by less powerful people; Lakoff, 1990). Meta-analyses have shown that even those gender differences that have been documented are generally small and becoming smaller over time (Hyde & Linn, 1986; Voyer, Voyer, & Bryden, 1995).

Focusing on gender differences often results in disregarding variations within each gender that are related to class, race, sexual orientation, and so forth. Conclusions about gender differences are often based on small, unrepresentative samples from the dominant group (e.g., primarily white, primarily middle or upper middle class, primarily heterosexual samples of U.S. college students). Some gender differences that hold for women and men of one race or sexual orientation do not hold for another (e.g., Koss, 1993, p. 204; Lott, 1990, p. 75). Nevertheless, often the experiences of the dominant group are universalized, and the experiences of nondominant groups are disregarded, resulting in a "homogenization of women's experience" (Rhode, 1990, p. 5). Furthermore, such approaches are typically ahistorical, based on the implicit assumption that gender differences are static over time and place (Rhode, 1990).

Finally, the differences approach has practical consequences. Because it gives inadequate attention to situational factors that produce gender differences, existing differences are viewed as innate and inevitable (Unger, 1990). Although both women's and men's opportunities have been restricted based on these assumptions, the differences approach has been especially detrimental to women's opportunities. The idea of separate spheres for women and men has been used to make women responsible for most of the housework, even though most women are also in the paid work force; this results in many women working a "second shift" (Hare-Mustin & Marecek, 1990; Hochschild, 1989). Some people consciously and overtly discriminate, arguing that women do not belong in certain jobs or roles. Others do not hold such overtly discriminatory views; nevertheless, they view certain jobs and roles as more appropriate for women and others as more appropriate for men. As a result, in this culture the preponderance of social, economic, and political power is held by men (Unger & Crawford, 1992). Furthermore, because "women's presumed differences from men are used to justify unequal treatment" (Hare-Mustin & Marecek, 1990, p. 38), this unequal treatment and unequal experience can create actual gender differences.

Focusing on gender differences harms men as well as women: It exacerbates men's fears of being seen as feminine, and thus it promotes conformity to male stereotypes (Hare-Mustin & Marecek, 1990). Conformity to these stereotypes restricts men's behavior, such as by making men feel compelled to achieve in the workplace and in sports, by distancing men from their children, and so forth (Farrell, 1993; Fasteau, 1975). Men's gender role conformity also harms women, such as by forcing women to undertake a disproportionate burden of caregiving to children and the elderly and leaving women vulnerable to men's violence.

## Theories Focusing on Gender Similarities

Other theories emphasize gender similarities. McFadden (1984) referred to theorists who emphasize gender similarities as *minimizers*. Hare-Mustin and Marecek (1990) referred to the minimization of gender differences as *beta bias*, based on beta, or Type II, errors, in which researchers conclude that there are no group differences when in fact there are. Beta bias, they wrote, occurs when one assumes that what is true for men is or should be true for women or when one ignores differences in the social or economic resources available to women and men or ignores differences in "the social meanings and consequences of their actions" (p. 35).

Focusing on gender similarities does not necessitate any one political stance (McFadden, 1984). At the conservative end of the continuum are those who assume that what is true for men is or should be true for women, such as those who advocate that, in the name of fairness, women should be treated as men are treated (e.g., if a company does not allow parental leave for new fathers, fairness dictates not allowing it for new mothers) and those who assume that what is true for men is true of people in general (e.g., medical research based on men can be applied to everyone). Feminist concepts of gender that focus on similarities include advocating that both women and men can have "feminine" and "masculine" traits (Bem, 1974) and advocating equal rights for women and men (e.g., a position supported in the United States by the National Organization for Women; McFadden, 1984). At the radical extreme of the gender-similarities continuum are those who want to abolish female pregnancy—and the resulting gender inequities—through technological means (Firestone, 1971).

### A Critique of Gender-Similarities Approaches

Gender-similarities approaches challenge the unwarranted stereotypes that proliferate in this culture. By focusing on gender similarities, however, feminists may "risk reinforcing a value structure they seek to challenge. Affirmations of similarity between women and men may inadvertently universalize or validate norms of the dominant social group, norms that have been inattentive to women's interests, experiences, and perspectives" (Rhode, 1990, p. 3). Along similar lines, Rush (1990) argued that gender neutrality is a strategy used in the backlash against feminism: "Gender neutrality is rooted in the idea that both genders, male and female, are equally oppressed and that any attempt to hold men and male institutions accountable for transgressions against women is no longer fashionable nor acceptable" (p. 170). Similarly, MacKinnon (1990) wrote that "gender neutrality means that you cannot take gender into account . . . neutrality enforces a non-neutral status quo" (p. 12).

Equal treatment under the law has increased women's opportunities in education and the workplace (Hare-Mustin & Marecek, 1990). In the name of equality, however, practices based on men's needs and experiences have been applied to women. Hewlett (1986) presented a devastating analysis of the economic and social problems that the equal-rights approach has caused for women in the United States in matters such as parental leave and no-fault divorce laws. Tavris (1992) described the problems caused for women—in areas ranging from research on life-threatening illnesses to waiting lines in public rest rooms—when gender equality is confused with gender sameness and when both women and men are treated according to standards developed to meet the needs of men.

## Approaches to Gender Not Based on the Difference–Similarity Question

There are other ways to conceptualize gender that do not revolve around the degree of difference between women and men. In these approaches, rather than denying or celebrating difference, "the objective is to dislodge difference as the exclusive focus of gender-related questions" (Rhode, 1990, p. 6).

Focusing on issues other than gender difference–similarity does not necessitate any one political stance. At the more conservative end of the political continuum is accepting the categories of female and male, women and men, but asking questions that do not compare women and men (e.g., investigating women's relationships with each other without focusing on how women's relationships compare with men's relationships). Another approach not focusing on gender difference–similarity would be investigating how gender interacts with other "power distributions that cut across sex-based categories" (Rhode, 1990, p. 6), such as race or sexual orientation.

At the radical end of this continuum is a social constructionist approach to gender. Social constructionism focuses on how meaning is negotiated and how the culture influences knowledge (Gergen, 1985). From a social constructionist perspective, "the terms in which the world is understood are social artifacts, products of historically situated interchanges among people" (Gergen, 1985, p. 267). Language structures people's experience and is thus an important resource controlled by those in power. A social constructionist position assumes that gender, rather than located within the individual, is situated in the culture. What gender means and what we know about gender is culturally constructed. There is no universal way to understand gender; instead, gender is a socially constructed phenomenon that is understood in different ways in different cultures.

Thus, from a social constructionist framework, it is not the case that the two genders are different or similar; it is not even the case that there are necessarily two genders. Social constructionists would not ask, How different are women and men? Instead, they would ask, How is gender constructed in this culture? What processes amplify or mute the significance of gender? Who benefits and who loses if we accept various theories of gender?

When asked where she stood on the maximalist–minimalist debate, Tavris (1992) decided that "the question itself is the problem" because "all polarities of thinking, like all dichotomies of groups, are by nature artificial, misleading, and oversimplified" (p. 288). She preferred to emphasize the influence of context on women's and men's behavior (e.g., the person's role) and gender as narrative (i.e., the stories women and men tell). She asked,

> Who benefits from the official theories and private stories we tell about presumed sex differences? Who pays? What are the consequences? Who gets the jobs and promotions? Who ends up doing the housework? If a woman wishes to believe that her problem is PMS or codependency rather than an abusive or

simply unresponsive husband, how does she benefit? How does she lose? If a man wishes to believe that a woman is naturally better at relationships, emotions, and caretaking, how does he benefit? How does he lose? If society promotes the view that women are less reliable than men because of their hormones and their pregnancies, what are the consequences for equity at work, in the law, in politics? (Tavris, 1992, p. 289)

The "fact" that there are two sexes—female and male—is typically seen as a biological reality, a fact of nature, beyond dispute. From a social constructionist perspective, however, even this "fact" can be challenged. Fausto-Sterling (1993–1994) argued that, biologically, people do not fall neatly into the categories "female" and "male": Some people have both ovarian and testicular tissue; others have ovaries but "male" external genitals or testes but "female" external genitals. "Advances" in medicine, such as surgery and hormone therapy, have been used to medically construct two and only two sexes. These "medical accomplishments can be read not as progress but as a mode of discipline. Hermaphrodites have unruly bodies. They do not fall naturally into a binary classification; only a surgical shoehorn can put them there" (p. 11). Thus, according to Fausto-Sterling, the existence of two sexes is not a biological fact but a cultural construction.

Bem has challenged the notion of two genders. In the 1970s, she had proposed the theory of androgyny, postulating that both women and men can have similar characteristics (Bem, 1974). Nevertheless, she was frustrated by people's tendency to continue to divide the world into masculine and feminine (e.g., girls' toys and boys' toys; women's jobs and men's jobs). Recently, Bem (1995) proposed that rather than abandoning the concept of gender (in effect, reducing the number of genders from two to one), we could expand the number of genders. These genders would involve two biological sexes (female and male) crossed with three gender roles (masculine, feminine, and androgynous) crossed with three sexual orientations (heterosexual, homosexual, and bisexual); other dimensions could also be added. Bem's model was informed by evidence that when there are two categories, people tend to think in dichotomies (e.g., boys are athletic, girls are not; Barnes, 1984, cited in Deaux & Major, 1990); such dichotomization is less likely when there are three or more categories. Perhaps, Bem reasoned, having more than two genders would reduce the tendency to stereotype.

## A Critique of Approaches Not Based on the Difference–Similarity Question

Many of these approaches have the advantage of taking into consideration important categories other than gender, such as sexual orientation, race, class, and age, and how they interact with gender. Thus, they move away from a simplistic notion of gender in which white, middle-class, heterosexual women's and men's experiences are generalized to everyone, and they acknowledge that people have identities other than gender identities. These approaches also have the advantage of giving serious attention to situational factors that affect gendered behavior. The social constructionist perspective has the advantages of looking critically at the implicit, often unacknowledged, assumptions made about gender and of inquiring about the social and political impact of these assumptions.

These approaches highlight how ingrained our gender categories are and how difficult it is to move away from them. For example, even Bem's (1995) conceptualization included the categories "masculine" and "feminine," which imply that certain qualities are mainly associated with males and females. Even in this chapter, I use the words "women" and "men" and phrases such as "women's needs and experiences." Using these terms is convenient, but this convenience comes at a cost. These terms mask numerous differences among women and among men, and they imply commonalities within each gender that are often unwarranted (e.g., not all women have the same needs and experiences).

Clearly, the concept of gender is complex and the source of dispute. Acknowledging these complexities, I now turn specifically to the pros and cons of studying sexually aggressive women, keeping the following questions in mind: In what ways are researchers exhibiting alpha bias, unjustifiably treating women and men as opposites? In what ways are they exhibiting beta bias, overlooking important distinctions between women and men? What stories do they tell about gender differences in sexual aggression? Who benefits from these stories? Who loses?

# THE IMPORTANCE OF STUDYING SEXUALLY AGGRESSIVE WOMEN

## Avoiding Research Bias

Historically, social scientists have used gender stereotypes to guide sample selection; for example, studies on aggression have been done mostly on men, and studies on affiliation and social influence have been done mostly on women (McHugh, Keoske, & Frieze, 1986; Unger, 1990). "Some psychological researchers have used single-sex samples out of an erroneous belief that certain topics are only relevant to one sex" (McHugh et al., 1986, p. 885). One cannot draw conclusions about gender differences by "studying only one sex and then claiming how the other sex might differ if studied by the same approach" (Hare-Mustin & Marecek, 1990, p. 13). Denmark, Russo, Frieze, and Sechzer (1988), summarizing some of the ways sexism can influence psychological research, included "the selection of research participants . . . based on stereotypic assumptions" (p. 583). They recommended that "both sexes should be studied before conclusions are drawn" (p. 583). Only by studying both women and men can we draw informed conclusions about women's and men's rates of being sexually victimized or victimizing others and about the consequences and meanings of sexual aggression for women and men.

## Challenging Gender Stereotypes

Limiting research to studying only sexually aggressive men and the women they victimize implicitly perpetuates gender stereotypes, such as the stereotypes of men as active and women as passive, men as victimizers and women as victims, and men as always seeking sex[1] and women as either resisting or acquiescing to male pursuit. Such stereotypes reflect an alpha bias, exaggerating the differences between women and men.

---

[1]Despite the common saying, "Rape is violence, not sex," I am conceptualizing sexual aggression as related to sex (see Muehlenhard, Danoff-Burg, & Powch, 1996, for further discussion).

Two gender stereotypes that are specifically challenged by studying sexually aggressive women involve women's sexual passivity and men's sexual insatiability. "The perception of women's sexuality as less powerful, less compelling, and less profound than that of men is still almost universal" (Chalker, 1994, p. 1). Popular songs, advertising, advice columns, and even scientific texts typically portray men's sexuality as active, powerful, and unstoppable, while portraying women's sexuality as passive, responsive, and receptive (Martin, 1991; Reinholtz, Muehlenhard, Phelps, & Satterfield, 1995). Social scientists contribute to this discourse. If we study only sexually aggressive men and sexually victimized women, we implicitly support these stereotypes. If we study sexually aggressive women, we challenge these stereotypes. Documenting women who actively, even aggressively, seek sex could contribute to the discourse about women's sexual agency. Enhancing women's sexual agency could benefit women by giving them greater permission to initiate sex rather than waiting passively for their partners to initiate; it could benefit men by relieving them of the sole responsibility for sexual initiation. Conversely, documenting men who find women's sexual advances unwelcome could counter the prevailing discourse about men's sexual insatiability. Countering this stereotype could benefit men by making it easier for them to refuse unwanted sex; it could benefit women to the extent that some men sexually aggress against women in response to pressures to be sexually active (Kanin, 1967).

## Acknowledging Victims' Experiences

Ignoring sexually aggressive women ignores the harm they cause to victims, whether male or female, and could even exacerbate victims' distress by implying that their experiences are invalid or trivial. Victims of women's aggression may not report the violence in part because of "lack of perceived seriousness, or fear of being stigmatized" (White & Kowalski, 1994, pp. 490–491). Consistent with White and Kowalski's contention, an incident of a woman's sexual aggression against another woman recently appeared in a newspaper humor column, "News of the Weird" (1995). How likely is someone to tell others, or even to take their own experience seriously, if their experiences are the fodder of humor columns?

Although sexually aggressive women cause harm to both female and male victims, some consequences are specific to female or male victims.

## Female Victims

Focusing only on male perpetrators ignores sexual aggression that occurs within lesbian relationships (Waterman, Dawson, & Bologna, 1989). Lesbians victimized by their partners may feel as if their experiences are not validated.

There are numerous factors that contribute to the invisibility of sexual aggression in lesbian relationships. In this culture, penile–vaginal intercourse is often considered the only real form of sex (Chalker, 1994), and, as mentioned, violence perpetrated by women is often discounted as less serious than violence perpetrated by men (White & Kowalski, 1994). If lesbians cannot engage in "real" sex or "real" aggression, by extension, they cannot engage in "real" sexual aggression. In response to homophobia, lesbians may be defensive about admitting that sexual aggression exists within the lesbian community; they may be reluctant to challenge "the lesbian myth of healthy, violence-free, egalitarian relationships" (Coleman, 1994, p. 139). This reluctance is understandable, but it could deprive sexually victimized lesbians of community support. Research on sexual aggression in lesbian relationships could help to counter all these sources of invisibility. Research could also lead to greater understanding of the causes, consequences, and prevention of sexual aggression within lesbian relationships and could document the need for support services for sexually victimized lesbians (Waterman et al., 1989).

In addition to acknowledging individual lesbian victims, research on lesbian sexual aggression could contribute to the acknowledgment of lesbianism. Although there are some indications of change, in the U.S. culture lesbianism is often invisible (Rich, 1980). This invisibility leads to what Rich (1980) called "compulsory heterosexuality": Heterosexuality is presented as women's only option. Studying sexual aggression within lesbian relationships could contribute to the visibility of lesbian relationships.

## Male Victims

Women's sexual coercion of men has often been treated less than seriously. Humor columnist Suzanne Fields (1988) satirized a study in which male Texas A&M University students ("Aggies") reported engaging in unwanted sex. The article began, "Alas, there is bad news for Southern macho from College Station, where a Texas Aggie in a pickup, with a six-pack in his belly and a Lone Star can crushed in his fist, will never again be celebrated for mucho macho. One of those ubiquitous studies, this one a study of Aggieland, reveals that Aggies, of all people, are complaining that the Aggie women are making them do 'it' " (p. C7). The column continued in this vein. Even esteemed researchers have sometimes seemed to make light of the possibility of men's being sexually victimized by women. Koss (1988) wrote, "Under a sex neutral definition of rape, a woman could rape a man but this would involve acts such as a group of women forcibly holding a man down *while they use carrots* to penetrate him anally" (p. 191, emphasis added). Men themselves may be unable to see themselves as victimized, even when they are victimized in the objective sense. Battered men must be more seriously injured than battered women before they perceive themselves as victims (Letellier, 1994); the same may be true for sexual aggression.

Studying women's sexual aggression against men could contribute to the understanding of the causes, consequences, and prevention of such aggression, and it could lead to a greater acknowledgment of this problem when it does occur. As Fields's satire demonstrates, however, the existence of research on men who are sexually coerced by women does not guarantee that the issue will be taken seriously. Perhaps more research documenting the negative consequences that some men experience would increase people's sensitivity, making jokes about sexually victimized men as socially unacceptable as jokes about sexually victimized women.

## Going Beyond Sexism to Acknowledge Other Forms of Oppression

Some writers have urged feminists to broaden our focus to address not only sexism but also other forms of oppression, such as racism, classism, heterosexism, and ageism (e.g., hooks, 1989/1995; Lorde,

1984). Such a broadened focus requires acknowledging the guilt-inducing fact that not only are women oppressed but women also oppress others. For example, a woman might oppress people of other races, people of other classes, or children (hooks, 1989/1995).

It is easy for women to think in terms of "us" and "them" regarding victimization, with women being "us," the victims, and men being "them," the victimizers. But, as bell hooks (1989/1995) wrote, "emphasizing paradigms of domination that call attention to woman's capacity to dominate is one way to deconstruct and challenge the simplistic notion that man is the enemy, woman the victim; the notion that men have always been the oppressors. Such thinking enables us to examine our role as woman in the perpetuation and maintenance of systems of domination" (p. 492). Examining our role in oppressing others is an essential first step to ending such oppression. Studying women's sexual aggressiveness is one area in which we can examine women's capacity to dominate others.

## Enriched Theories

Acknowledging sexually aggressive women could lead us to examine the limitations of existing theories that explain sexual aggression solely in terms of gender socialization, gender roles, and sexism. Studying sexually aggressive women could lead to richer, more complex theories. Numerous other variables may be important in explaining sexual aggression. The following variables have been suggested as worth consideration in explaining battering; they may also be important for sexual aggression: sexual orientation, homophobia, and heterosexism; race and racism; social class and classism; age and ageism; personality and psychopathology; developmental, neurological, and physiological variables; economic and political factors; social stress; social isolation; family dynamics; community-related variables; cultural beliefs; how people conceptualize and respond to violence; how violence is used to maintain power and control over a partner separate from gender; and possible interactions among all these variables (Coleman, 1994; Letellier, 1994; Miller, 1994; Renzetti, 1994). Clearly, violent relationships and aggressors are not monolithic; complex theories can take more of this variability into account.

An example of the value of moving beyond gender alone as an

explanatory variable can be seen in a study by Brenner (1994). She investigated the effects of both gender and a history of childhood sexual abuse on the likelihood of subsequently being sexually coerced and sexually coercing others (in this study, "sexual coercion" included both verbal and physical sexual coercion). Brenner found main effects for gender such that more women (52.5%) than men (23.3%) had been sexually coerced as adolescents or adults, and more men (32.5%) than women (7.9%) had sexually coerced other adolescents or adults. Those women and men who had been sexually abused as children were more likely than those who had not to report having been sexually coerced as adolescents and adults (47.5% vs. 35.8%, respectively) and to report having sexually coerced other adolescents or adults (27.6% vs. 18.2%). Having been sexually abused as a child increased the likelihood of being sexually coerced as an adolescent or adult—and increased the likelihood of sexually coercing others—similarly for women and men. Clearly, gender was an important variable in predicting sexual coercion, but it was not the only important variable.

## Toward Prevention

Studying sexual aggression and identifying its causes could contribute to preventing women's sexual aggression against both women and men. Paradoxically, it could also contribute to preventing men's sexual aggression. Research suggests that when women are sexually aggressive, they are usually less physically forceful than are men (e.g., Muehlenhard & Long, 1988). If even this less physically forceful type of sexual aggression were considered unacceptable, this could be a good model for everyone—both women and men—to follow. Trivializing women's sexual aggression may result in rationalizing and trivializing similar behavior when it is engaged in by men; taking both women's and men's sexual aggression seriously is preferable.

# THE DANGER OF STUDYING SEXUALLY AGGRESSIVE WOMEN

## The Danger of Gender Neutrality

Despite its importance, studying sexually aggressive women, and thereby acknowledging that both men and women can be perpetrators, could lead to beta bias, in which important gender differences are minimized. Studying sexually aggressive women is problematic if it implies that gender is irrelevant to sexual coercion or that sexual coercion is a gender-neutral problem. As discussed previously, gender neutrality can perpetuate the status quo and strengthen systems in which women must conform to standards based on the experiences, needs, and abilities of men. In this section, I discuss some of the areas in which gender plays a role in sexual aggression.

## Gender Differences in the Likelihood of Being a Victim or Perpetrator

More women than men are sexually victimized by others[2] (e.g., Brenner, 1994; Koss, 1993). In a recent study of 3,432 women and men, ages 18 to 59, drawn from randomly selected geographic areas across the United States, 22% of the women compared with 2% of the men indicated that they had been forced to do something sexually (Michael, Gagnon, Laumann, & Kolata, 1994). Of the men who reported being forced, one-third reported being forced by another man; two-thirds reported being forced by a woman. Of the women who reported being forced, 99.4% reported being forced by a man; only 0.6% reported being forced by a woman. "Three percent of men report having forced a woman and two-tenths of a percent say they forced a man," whereas "only a minuscule proportion of women say they ever forced a woman or a man" (Michael et al., 1994, p. 227). Thus, the overwhelming majority of forced sex involves men forcing women, but studying women as aggressors may obscure this fact.

## Gender Differences in Fear and Loss of Freedom

Women consistently report being more afraid of rape than men do, and women restrict their behavior more than men do (Gordon & Riger, 1989). Gordon and Riger interviewed women and men in

---

[2]An exception to this general conclusion involves gay men and lesbians; more gay men than lesbians report having been sexually assaulted (Koss, 1993). Thus, just as a simplistic gender-similarities approach is inadequate, a simplistic gender-differences approach is likewise inadequate. We need to go beyond mere gender differences or similarities to a more complex view of the problem.

three large U.S. cities. The interviews included questions about their fears and self-protective behaviors. They found that self-protective behaviors comprised (or, in statistical terms, loaded on) two general factors: "street smarts" and isolation. Women engaged in both types of behaviors more often than men did. For example, 73.9% of the women, compared with 29.4% of the men, reported that they "often" used street smarts to keep themselves safe, such as wearing shoes that permitted them to run in case of danger, choosing bus or movie seats with an eye toward who would be sitting nearby, avoiding looking strangers in the eye, and avoiding dressing in a sexy manner. Furthermore, 41.5% of the women, compared with 10.3% of the men, reported that they "often" isolated themselves, going out only in the daytime and avoiding doing errands and activities that they wanted to do, because they feared for their safety. Significantly more women than men reported (Gordon & Riger, 1989, p. 15) that they

- Never walked in their neighborhoods alone after dark (25.3% of the women vs. 2.9% of the men).
- Never went to movies alone after dark (74.9% vs. 32.4%).
- Never went to bars or clubs alone after dark (68.4% vs. 5.4%).
- Never used public transit alone after dark (46.3% vs. 29.4%).
- Never went downtown alone after dark (47.0% vs. 7.5%).
- Never walked by parks or empty lots alone after dark (52.8% vs. 13.2%).

The picture that emerges is one of many women virtually imprisoned inside their homes at night and preoccupied with keeping themselves safe if they do go out. This picture is not gender-neutral: Overwhelmingly, it is women who bear the burden of fear of being raped.

Not surprisingly, when women fear being raped, they fear being raped by men, not other women. In a study in which women were asked gender-neutral questions about their fears of rape (e.g., "What types of situations/circumstances, if any, make you afraid of being raped by someone you know/don't know?"), the women mentioned numerous situations in which they were afraid of men but none in which they were afraid of women (Hickman & Muehlenhard, 1997).

## Gender Differences in Force and Consent

Gender influences the meaning of force. In defining rape, most legal reform statutes are gender-neutral, applying the same concept of forced sex to women and men (Estrich, 1987). Nevertheless, the concept of force is not gender-neutral (Estrich, 1987). Because of differences between women's and men's size, strength, and socialization, usually less force is needed to overcome women than men. Because of these differences, applying a gender-neutral standard to forced sex, in which women are expected to have the same ability as men to resist rape, is unjust to women: "Gender neutrality suggests that rape law can be made and enforced without regard to the different ways men and women understand force and consent. That might work if the governing standard were defined by the understanding of most women. But all experience suggests that if there is only one standard, it will be a male standard" (Estrich, 1987, p. 82). And in fact, the legal standard typically has been a male standard. Estrich reviewed rape and sexual assault laws and appellate court decisions that required women to use physical resistance to demonstrate their lack of consent, sometimes requiring of women the "utmost resistance." In many of these cases, judges expected women to fight: "Their version of a reasonable person is one who does not scare easily, one who does not feel vulnerable, one who is not passive, one who fights back, not cries. The reasonable woman, it seems, is not a schoolboy 'sissy'; she is a real man" (Estrich, 1987, p. 65). Estrich concluded that legally, gender neutrality is unfair to women: "Sometimes the failure to discriminate is discriminatory; where there are real differences, failure to recognize and take account of them is the proof of unfairness" (Estrich, 1987, p. 25).

Gender may also influence the meaning of "consenting" to sex (Muehlenhard, Powch, Phelps, & Giusti, 1992). For example, men generally make more money than do women, and wives are often economically dependent on their husbands. If a woman believes that refusing to have sex with her husband could lead to divorce, and divorce could lead to economic hardship, perhaps even homelessness (Liebow, 1993), what choice does she have but to "consent" to sex? "When material conditions preclude 99 percent of your options, it is not meaningful to call the remaining 1 percent—what you are doing—your choice . . . consent is not a meaningful concept" (MacKinnon, 1990, p. 4).

Some feminist theorists have argued that women can never freely consent to sex. For example, A Southern Women's Writing Collective (1990) argued that in this culture, women are taught to be sexually aroused by what men regard as sexual. Thus, if a woman feels aroused and thinks that she is consenting, this is only because cultural indoctrination has succeeded. Furthermore, they argued, in this culture sex is part of a "package" including sex, love, companionship, and economic support; rejecting sex leads to losing all these. As long as this is the case, they argued, sex in this culture can never be truly voluntary for any woman.

Men as well as women face cultural indoctrination about their expected sexual behavior. Our culture is dominated by men (e.g., all U.S. presidents and most senators and representatives, CEOs of powerful corporations, religious leaders, etc., have been men; e.g., Cassata, 1994). Nevertheless, any one man rejecting the dominant culture's construction of male sexuality would face a considerable challenge. For men, there may be little social support for refusing sex (Beneke, 1982; Muehlenhard & Cook, 1988). Thus, women and men are similar in facing cultural indoctrination about sex, yet they are different in the particulars of that indoctrination.

## Gender Differences in the Meanings and Consequences of Sexual Aggression

The same set of objective events does not have one and only one meaning. People give meaning to the events they experience based on numerous circumstances, characteristics, and perspectives that they bring to the event: "The events we experience in our everyday lives do not have a 'given' meaning; the reality of our experience is a narrative reality; we respond not to the so-called 'objective' qualities of the perceived world, but to qualities that are a function of our *perspective upon* the world of experience" (Churchill, 1993, p. 21, emphasis in the original).

There is empirical evidence that sexual coercion has different meanings and consequences for women and men. For example, when women and men were asked identical questions about incidents in which someone did something sexual to them without their consent, there were many gender differences in their responses (Satterfield, 1995). Women and men differed in their reasons for not wanting to engage in the sexual activity: Women, more than men, reported that they had not wanted to engage in the activity because they were inexperienced or feared pregnancy, because it was too early in the relationship, because they were intoxicated, because the other person was someone they did not know or like, and because they were uninterested; there were no reasons that men reported more than women. In describing what actually compelled them to engage in the unwanted act, women, more than men, reported that they had been compelled by threats of violence or actual violence, by the other person's ignoring their refusals or proceeding without their consent, and by feelings of guilt if they refused; the only compelling factor that men reported more than women was peer pressure. Women, more than men, reported reacting to the incident with thoughts of confusion, anger, and self-blame; men, more than women, reported reacting to the incident with thoughts that the incident had been either inconsequential or fun. Finally, women, more than men, reported reacting to the incident with feelings of self- and other-directed negative emotions and depression; men, more than women, reported reacting to the incident with feelings of satisfaction and other positive feelings. Taken together, these differences suggest that incidents of sexual coercion do indeed have different meanings and consequences for women than for men (Satterfield, 1995). Other studies have also shown that women report being more distressed than men about having been sexually coerced (e.g., Muehlenhard & Long, 1988; Struckman-Johnson, 1988). Nevertheless, it would be a mistake to overgeneralize. For example, Satterfield (1995) found that for all of these consequences, there were overlaps among women's and men's responses; that is, some men reported being more distressed than did some women.

Reasons for these differences are probably varied. One reason could be gender differences in the meaning of sex. Tiefer (1995) argued that "men and women are raised with different sets of sexual values—men toward varied experience and physical gratification, women toward intimacy and emotional communication" (p. 55). To the extent a man and woman hold such values, sexual aggression may be less negative for him than for her, because sexual aggression may still meet his need for varied sexual experience and physical gratification while not meeting her need for intimacy and emotional communication.

There still exists a sexual double standard in which sex is regarded as enhancing men's status but diminishing women's status

(Muehlenhard & McCoy, 1991; Tiefer, 1995). A sexually active man may be called a "stud" whereas a sexually active woman may be called a "slut." Furthermore, "within women's ascribed roles as unequals, sex is something that women give to men" (Miller, cited in Amaro, 1995, p. 443). To the extent that a man and woman believe that men win and women lose through sex, it is understandable that sexual aggression may be more devastating to her than to him even if their objective circumstances are the same.

Sex, and thus sexual aggression, could also have different meanings to women and men for other reasons: Women lack secure reproductive rights. Women are more likely than men to have psychological scars from sexual abuse (Tiefer, 1995). Male-to-female transmission of sexually transmitted diseases is 12 times more likely than female-to-male transmission (Padian, Shiboski, & Jewell, 1990, cited in Amaro, 1995).

Koss (1993) argued that having one's body penetrated is crucial to the meaning of sexual coercion. Thus, she declared that when defining rape and studying its prevalence, it would be incorrect merely to ask women and men about their experiences with being coerced into unwanted sexual intercourse. Even if a man is forced to engage in sexual intercourse with a woman, this would not be rape because the man was not being penetrated: "If men and boys are to be included, care must be taken to ensure that their data are accurate counterparts of rape prevalence among women. This means that [to be counted as rape victims] men must be reporting instances where they experienced penetration of their own body (or attempts)" (Koss, 1993, p. 218). Thus, based on Koss's argument, women may react to sexual aggression more negatively than do men because women are more likely than men to experience sexual penetration of their bodies.

There is empirical support for the idea that sexual penetration is more traumatic than nonpenetrative sex acts. In a study of child sexual abuse, Russell (1986, pp. 99 and 143) found that among women who had, as children, experienced completed or attempted sexual penetration (i.e., intercourse, fellatio, cunnilingus, analingus, or anal intercourse), 54% later said that they were extremely traumatized. This percentage compares with 35% of the women who had, as children, experienced touching of their unclothed breasts or genitals and 19% of those who had experienced kissing or touching of their clothed breasts or genitals. Thus, sexual penetration was generally associated with greater trauma than was being touched.

Nevertheless, in noting the differences between women's and men's experiences, it is important that we do not portray women and men as opposites. Even though there are numerous statistically significant gender differences in women's and men's reactions to sexual aggression, studies still show considerable overlap in the responses of women and men (Muehlenhard & Long, 1988; Satterfield, 1995), with some men being more upset than some women. Some women and men espouse the sexual double standard, but others do not. There is no one-to-one correspondence between a sexual act and its meaning or consequences: Russell (1986) found that some women who had experienced sexual penetration reported that they had not been extremely traumatized, whereas other women who had experienced nonpenetrative acts reported that they had been extremely traumatized. Similarly, we cannot assume that forced intercourse or oral sex is less traumatic to a man than to a woman just because he was not penetrated. Consequences of sexual aggression are affected by the complex meanings that people bring to it.

## Potential for Backlash against Feminist Activism

Studying sexually aggressive women could be used as fuel for the backlash against feminist activists working to end violence against women. Some women's groups have resisted research on aggressive women, fearing it "would draw attention away from men's far more lethal aggression" (Campbell, 1993, p. 143). Research on women's aggression could fuel the backlash if critics argue that feminism is making women aggressive (White & Kowalski, 1994). Findings of sexual violence in lesbian relationships could fuel attacks on lesbianism.

The pattern here could replicate what happened with research on battering. In 1978, Suzanne Steinmetz published an article stating that husbands were also victims of domestic violence and that husband abuse was even more underreported than wife abuse. In the uproar that followed, some opponents of the women's movement used these findings to argue against funding shelters for battered women (see Gelles & Straus, 1988). Subsequent studies have shown that battered wives report more injuries than do battered husbands. Furthermore, violent wives typically report self-defense or retaliatory reasons for their violence, whereas violent husbands more often report external or situational factors or coercive and controlling reasons (Hamberger & Potente, 1994; White & Kowalski, 1994). Prevalence statistics alone did not take these factors into account, however, and they provided fuel for a backlash.

Along similar lines, it is possible that research on women's sexual aggression could be used by opponents of rape crisis centers or rape prevention programs to decrease funding. This in itself probably should not be enough to argue against such research; there is little research that cannot be distorted and used against women. In fact, Neil Gilbert (1991, 1993), a professor and antifeminist activist, has already distorted Koss's and Russell's research on men's sexual assault against women; he used his distortions to argue against funding rape crisis centers "to combat an epidemic that does not exist" (Gilbert, 1993, p. A18). He did not need research on women's sexual aggression against men to fuel his arguments (see Muehlenhard, Sympson, Phelps, & Highby, 1994, for further discussion). Nevertheless, in conceptualizing studies on sexually aggressive women and in interpreting the results, researchers should be aware of the potential for backlash.

## Misdirected Resources

Another danger of studying sexually aggressive women could be that, if sexual coercion is seen as a gender-neutral problem, resources might be misdirected. Equal resources might be allocated to prevention programs aimed at male and female perpetrators. As we have seen, sexual coercion is not a gender-neutral problem. Although it would be reasonable to allocate some funds to prevention programs aimed at female perpetrators, a reasonable allocation would involve greater attention to male than to female perpetrators.

## RECOMMENDATIONS AND CONCLUSIONS

Based on consideration of these issues, I recommend the following:

1. To account for sexually aggressive women, we need to revise theories that are based solely on gender socialization, gender

roles, and sexism. We should consider numerous other variables that might enrich our theories: sexual orientation, race and ethnicity, class, age, personality and psychopathology, and so forth.

2. Nevertheless, we should not ignore gender as a variable. There is overwhelming evidence that sexual aggression is not gender-neutral in its prevalence, in the fear and life restrictions that it induces, or in its meanings and consequences. Research on sexually aggressive women should be sensitive to the influence of gender on all aspects of respondents' experiences.

3. Be careful when using parallel terms and concepts for women and men. A given term or concept (e.g., force) may have different meanings to women and men.

4. Remember that sexual aggressors and victims are not monolithic groups. No one explanation will allow us to understand every situation.

5. Researchers should be sensitive to the potential that their results could be used to fuel the backlash against antiviolence programs. Researchers should be careful about how they frame their questions and results, being sure to contextualize their findings and to compare women and men not only with respect to the frequency of sexually coercive events but also with respect to the meanings and consequences of these events.

6. Even when research reveals group differences, "at the individual case level, a careful assessment must be conducted to determine whether the situation at hand fits the generalization or not" (Hamberger & Potente, 1994, p. 128).

Returning to the beginning of this chapter and the dinner conversation with my fellow researcher, I think we were both right. It is important to study female sexual aggression, but such an undertaking is not simple and is not without risk. These issues go to the heart of the meaning of gender. Neither emphasizing gender similarities nor emphasizing gender differences has solely positive or negative ramifications. It is important to go beyond gender alone and look at other variables that may interact with gender. And it is important to ask who benefits and who loses from how we approach these issues.

## REFERENCES

A Southern Women's Writing Collective. (1990). Sex resistance in hetero-sexual arrangements. In D. Leidholdt & J. Raymond (Eds.), *The sexual liberals and the attack on feminism* (pp. 140–147). New York: Pergamon.

Alaimo, S. (1994). Cyborg and ecofeminist interventions: Challenges for an environmental feminism. *Feminist Studies, 20,* 133–152.

Amaro, H. (1995). Love, sex, and power: Considering women's realities in HIV prevention. *American Psychologist, 50,* 437–447.

Andelin, H. B. (1980). *Fascinating womanhood.* New York: Bantam.

Bem, S. L. (1974). The measurement of psychological androgyny. *Journal of Consulting and Clinical Psychology, 42,* 155–162.

Bem, S. L. (1995). Dismantling gender polarization and compulsory heterosexuality: Should we turn the volume down or up? *Journal of Sex Research, 32,* 329–334.

Beneke, T. (1982). *Men on rape.* New York: St. Martin's Press.

Brenner, L. M. (1994). *The adult patterns of men and women who were sexually abused as children: Is there risk of becoming a victim or perpetrator?* Unpublished doctoral dissertation, University of Kansas, Lawrence.

Broverman, I. K., Vogel, S. R., Broverman, D. M., Clarkson, F. E., & Rosenkrantz, P. S. (1972). Sex-role stereotypes: A current appraisal. *Journal of Social Issues, 28,* 59–78.

Campbell, A. (1993). *Men, women, and aggression.* New York: Basic Books.

Cassata, D. (1994, November 12). Freshman class boasts resumes to back up "outsider" image. *Congressional Quarterly, 52*(44, Suppl.), 9–12.

Chalker, R. (1994). Updating the model of female sexuality. *SIECUS Report, 22,* 1–6.

Churchill, S. D. (1993). The lived meanings of date rape: Seeing through the eyes of the victim. *Family Violence and Sexual Assault Bulletin, 9,* 20–23.

Colby, A., & Damon, W. (1987). Listening to a different moral voice: A review of Gilligan's *In a Different Voice.* In M. R. Walsh (Ed.), *The psychology of women: Ongoing debates* (pp. 321–329). New Haven, CT: Yale University Press.

Coleman, V. E. (1994). Lesbian battering: The relationship between personality and the perpetration of violence. *Violence and Victims, 9,* 139–152.

Deaux, K., & Major, B. (1990). A social-psychological model of gender. In D. L. Rhode (Ed.), *Theoretical perspectives on sexual difference* (pp. 89–99). New Haven, CT: Yale University Press.

Denmark, F., Russo, N. F., Frieze, I. H., & Sechzer, J. A. (1988).

Guidelines for avoiding sexism in psychological research: A report of the Ad Hoc Committee on Nonsexist Research. *American Psychologist, 43,* 582–585.

Estrich, S. (1987). *Real rape.* Cambridge, MA: Harvard University Press.

Farrell, W. (1993). *The myth of male power: Why men are the disposable sex.* New York: Simon & Schuster.

Fasteau, M. F. (1975). *The male machine.* New York: Dell.

Fausto-Sterling, A. (1993–1994). The five sexes: Why male and female are not enough. *Journal of Gender Studies, 15–16,* 5–13.

Fields, S. (1988, December 20). Macho Aggie image shattered in college survey of sex lives. *Austin American-Statesman,* p. C7.

Firestone, S. (1971). *The dialectic of sex: The case for feminist revolution.* New York: Bantam.

Gelles, R. J., & Straus, M. A. (1988). *Intimate violence.* New York: Simon & Schuster.

Gergen, K. J. (1985). The social constructionist movement in modern psychology. *American Psychologist, 40,* 266–275.

Gilbert, N. (1991). The phantom epidemic of sexual assault. *Public Interest, 103,* 54–65.

Gilbert, N. (1993, June 29). The wrong response to rape. *Wall Street Journal,* p. A18.

Gilligan, C. (1982). *In a different voice: Psychological theory and women's development.* Cambridge, MA: Harvard University Press.

Gordon, M. T., & Riger, S. (1989). *The female fear.* New York: Free Press.

Gray, J. (1994). *Men are from Mars; women are from Venus.* New York: HarperCollins.

Hamberger, L. K., & Potente, T. (1994). Counseling heterosexual women arrested for domestic violence: Implications for theory and practice. *Violence and Victims, 9,* 125–137.

Hare-Mustin, R. T., & Marecek, J. (Eds.). (1990). *Making a difference: Psychology and the construction of gender.* New Haven, CT: Yale University Press.

Hewlett, S. A. (1986). *A lesser life: The myth of women's liberation in America.* New York: William Morrow.

Hickman, S. E., & Muehlenhard, C. L. (1997). College women's fears and precautionary behaviors relating to acquaintance rape and stranger rape. *Psychology of Women Quarterly, 21,* 527–547.

Hoagland, S. L., & Penelope, J. (1988). *For lesbians only: A separatist anthology.* London: Onlywomen Press.

Hochschild, A. R. (1989). *The second shift.* New York: Basic Books.

hooks, b. (1995). Feminism: A transformational politic. In P. S. Rothenberg (Ed.), *Race, class, and gender in the United States: An integrated study* (3rd ed., pp. 491–498). New York: St. Martin's Press. (Excerpted from hooks, b., 1989, *Talking back: Thinking feminist, thinking Black,* Boston: South End Press)

Hyde, J. S., & Linn, M. C. (Eds.). (1986). *The psychology of gender: Advances through meta-analysis.* Baltimore: Johns Hopkins University.

Kanin, E. J. (1967). Reference groups and sex conduct norm violations. *Sociological Quarterly, 8,* 495–504.

Koss, M. P. (1988). Afterword: The methods used in the *Ms.* project on campus sexual assault. In R. Warshaw (Ed.), *I never called it rape* (pp. 189–210). New York: Harper & Row.

Koss, M. P. (1993). Detecting the scope of rape: A review of prevalence research methods. *Journal of Interpersonal Violence, 8,* 198–222.

Lakoff, R. T. (1990). *Talking power: The politics of language.* New York: Basic Books.

Letellier, P. (1994). Gay and bisexual male domestic violence victimization: Challenges to feminist theory and responses to violence. *Violence and Victims, 9,* 95–106.

Liebow, E. (1993). *Tell them who I am: The lives of homeless women.* New York: Free Press.

Lorde, A. (1984). *Sister outsider.* Freedom, CA: Crossing Press.

Lott, B. (1990). Dual nature of learned behavior: The challenge to feminist psychology. In R. T. Hare-Mustin & J. Marecek (Eds.), *Making a difference: Psychology and the construction of gender* (pp. 65–101). New Haven, CT: Yale University Press.

MacKinnon, C. A. (1990). Liberalism and the death of feminism. In D. Leidholdt & J. G. Raymond (Eds.), *The sexual liberals and the attack on feminism* (pp. 3–13). New York: Pergamon.

Martin, E. (1991). The egg and the sperm: How science has constructed a romance based on stereotypical male–female roles. *Signs: Journal of Women in Culture and Society, 16,* 485–501.

McFadden, M. (1984). Anatomy of difference: Toward a classification of feminist theory. *Women's Studies International Forum, 7,* 495–504.

McHugh, M. C., Keoske, R. D., & Frieze, I. H. (1986). Issues to consider in conducting nonsexist psychological research: A guide for researchers. *American Psychologist, 41,* 879–890.

Michael, R. T., Gagnon, J. H., Laumann, E. O., & Kolata, G. (1994). *Sex in America: A definitive survey.* Boston: Little, Brown.

Miller, S. L. (1994). Extending the boundaries: Toward a more inclusive and integrated study of intimate violence. *Violence and Victims, 9,* 183–194.

Morawski, J. G. (1987). The troubled quest for masculinity, femininity, and androgyny. In P. Shaver & C. Hendrick (Eds.), *Sex and gender* (pp. 44–69). Newbury Park, CA: Sage.

Muehlenhard, C. L., & Cook, S. W. (1988). Men's self-reports of unwanted sexual activity. *Journal of Sex Research, 24,* 58–72.

Muehlenhard, C. L., Danoff-Burg, S., & Powch, I. G. (1996). Is rape sex or violence? Conceptual issues and implications. In D. M. Buss & N. Malamuth (Eds.), *Sex, power, conflict: Feminist and evolutionary perspectives* (pp. 119–137). New York: Oxford University Press.

Muehlenhard, C. L., & Long, P. J. (1988, March). *Men's versus women's reports of pressure to engage in unwanted sexual intercourse.* Paper presented at the Western Region meeting of the Society for the Scientific Study of Sex, Dallas.

Muehlenhard, C. L., & McCoy, M. L. (1991). Double standard/double bind: The sexual double standard and women's communication about sex. *Psychology of Women Quarterly, 15,* 447–461.

Muehlenhard, C. L., Powch, I. G., Phelps, J. L., & Giusti, L. M. (1992). Definitions of rape: Scientific and political implications. *Journal of Social Issues, 48,* 23–44.

Muehlenhard, C. L., Sympson, S. C., Phelps, J. L., & Highby, B. J. (1994). Are rape statistics exaggerated? A response to criticism of contemporary rape research. *Journal of Sex Research, 31,* 134–136.

News of the weird. (1995, February 2). *University Daily Kansan,* p. 8A.

Reinholtz, R. K., Muehlenhard, C. L., Phelps, J. L., & Satterfield, A. T. (1995). Sexual discourse and sexual intercourse: How the way we communicate affects the way we think about sexual coercion. In P. J. Kalbfleisch & M. J. Cody (Eds.), *Gender, power and communication in human relationships* (pp. 141–162). Hillsdale, NJ: Erlbaum.

Renzetti, C. M. (1994). On dancing with a bear: Reflections on some of the current debates among domestic violence theorists. *Violence and Victims, 9,* 195–200.

Rhode, D. L. (1990). Theoretical perspectives on sexual difference. In D. L. Rhode (Ed.), *Theoretical perspectives on sexual difference* (pp. 1–9). New Haven, CT: Yale University Press.

Rich, A. (1980). Compulsory heterosexuality and lesbian existence. *Signs: Journal of Women in Culture and Society, 5,* 631–660.

Rush, F. (1990). The many faces of backlash. In D. Leidholdt & J. Raymond (Eds.), *The sexual liberals and the attack on feminism* (pp. 165–174). New York: Pergamon.

Russell, D. E. H. (1986). *The secret trauma: Incest in the lives of girls and women.* New York: Basic Books.

Satterfield, A. T. (1995). *The meaning of sexual coercion: An exploratory study of women's and men's experiences.* Unpublished doctoral dissertation, University of Kansas, Lawrence.

Struckman-Johnson, C. (1988). Forced sex on dates: It happens to men, too. *Journal of Sex Research, 24,* 234–241.

Tavris, C. (1992). *The mismeasure of woman.* New York: Simon & Schuster.

Tiefer, L. (1995). *Sex is not a natural act and other essays.* Boulder, CO: Westview.

Unger, R. K. (1990). Imperfect reflections of reality: Psychology constructs gender. In R. T. Hare-Mustin & J. Marecek (Eds.), *Making a difference: Psychology and the construction of gender* (pp. 102–149). New Haven, CT: Yale University Press.

Unger, R., & Crawford, M. (1992). *Women and gender: A feminist perspective.* New York: McGraw-Hill.

Voyer, D., Voyer, S., & Bryden, M. P. (1995). Magnitude of sex differences in spatial abilities: A meta-analysis and consideration of critical variables. *Psychological Bulletin, 117,* 250–270.

Waterman, C. K., Dawson, L. J., & Bologna, M. J. (1989). Sexual coercion in gay male and lesbian relationships: Predictors and implications for support services. *Journal of Sex Research, 26,* 118–124.

White, J. W., & Kowalski, R. M. (1994). Deconstructing the myth of the nonaggressive woman: A feminist analysis. *Psychology of Women Quarterly, 18,* 487–508.

# 3

# Theories, Politics, and Sexual Coercion

## ELIZABETH RICE ALLGEIER
## JENNIFER C. LAMPING

Given the fact that empirical research has been conducted on the phenomenon of unwanted sexual contacts for decades, it is surprising how little we *really* know about this behavior. Legal factors, theoretical assumptions, and methodological flaws all seem to have contributed to obscuring rather than enlightening our understanding of sexual assault. In this chapter we provide a brief overview of changes in societal and legal responses to sexual assault and coercion. We identify further areas in which social and legal reform is needed. However, we devote most of this chapter to a focus on the ways in which social scientists' strongly held beliefs and constructs are related to the questions we ask, how we ask them, and how we conduct our data analyses and interpret our findings. Our purpose in doing so is to encourage research that accurately reflects the interpersonal dynamics and judgments relevant to sexual assault so as to obtain information that can reduce the likelihood of coercive relationships and revictimization—regardless of victims' gender. We think that it is possible to reconcile our belief systems and our research activities so that neither is badly compromised, but only if, as Ira Reiss (1993) has written in a somewhat different context, we are aware of the potential impact of our beliefs on how we frame our research questions and interpret our findings. Reiss argued that it is impossible for us to be value-free. But to the extent that we are *aware* of our values and their contribution to the way in which we frame our research questions, we may be able to obtain more accurate answers regarding the phenomena we study (Reiss, 1993).

The judicial system's definitions of sexual assault have varied over the years, and even contemporary legal definitions may contribute to our confusion regarding the coercion of one person by another to engage in unwanted sex. Thus, we first review the varying legal definitions of sexual assault and the role that political activists have played in altering the definitions.

## POLITICS AND "RAPE" ADJUDICATION

Political activities aimed at protecting (primarily) women who report to legal authorities their alleged sexual assaults have resulted in major reforms in the ways in which charges of sexual assault are handled by members of the state judicial systems in the United States. Advocacy for such changes, designed to protect victims from further humiliation by the courts, has presumably been aided by the results of empirical work on sexual assault conducted by social scientists. In the process of addressing legal maltreatment of women victims, however, male victims of sexual coercion and assault have received very little attention. Further, in recent years, some political advocates and some social scientists have demonstrated hostility toward the idea that we should even be concerned with raped men's well-being. Some of this resistance is fueled by concerns that examination of men's and boys' potential victimization at the hands of the judicial system will reduce efforts to protect female victims—as one prominent self-described "feminist scholar" put it, such efforts will "undermine the feminist agenda."

## RAPE LAWS AND THE SOCIAL CONCEPTION OF SEXUAL AGGRESSION

Historically, laws governing rape have been narrowly defined and were consistent with stereotypic assumptions about sexual aggression held by laypeople, professionals, and researchers. In contrast, more recent laws have included a broader range of assaultive behaviors and expanded the original conception of rape. Even with these contemporary, more inclusive laws and conceptions, social stereotypes die hard.

Traditionally, rape laws in the United States mirrored English common law. That is, rape was defined as "illicit carnal knowledge of a female by force and against her will" (Black, 1968). This definition of rape in the legal and popular sphere was sustained until the beginning of the contemporary women's movement in the latter part of this century. According to the earlier conception, there were four necessary conditions for a particular behavior to be considered rape: (1) it had to be gender-specific, (2) it had to be extramarital, (3) it had to involve penetration of the vagina by the penis, and (4) it had to be forcible (Dixon, 1991). Thus, any type of sexual aggression falling outside the boundaries of these conditions (e.g., homosexual rape, marital rape, nonpenetrative rape, rapes of males by females, etc.) were not punishable by the law. In addition, under these traditional rape laws, convictions for perpetrators were elusive. It was necessary for victims to have substantive evidence as proof of the sexually assaultive event. For example, the victim either had to provide a witness or had to personally corroborate the identity of the perpetrator, the fact of penetration, and a lack of consent with much physical evidence (e.g., body bruises, torn clothing, vaginal tears, pregnancy, etc.). Finally, prior sexual history of the victim was permissible evidence used by the defense to discredit the victim or to establish that the activity was consensual (Dixon, 1991).

With the start of the contemporary women's movement in the 1960s and 1970s, many laws in the United States, including rape laws, were broadened. Rather than mandating national rape laws, states were given the liberty to draft their own version of laws to deal with sexual aggression. Although some adopted the narrowly defined, traditional laws, others adopted the traditional laws and made liberal amendments, and nearly half the states repealed the traditional definition of rape in favor of a new liberalized sexual assault law.

In contrast to traditional rape laws that focused on the institutional, gender-specific (male perpetrator/female victim), and sexual nature of the crime, liberalized sexual assault laws placed greater emphasis on the individual, gender-neutral, and violent nature of sexual coercion. Specifically, under contemporary assault law, coercion was defined as force or threat of force that violates human rights (Dixon, 1991). Thus, based on liberal laws, forced sexual contact was viewed as a crime punishable under the umbrella of assault rather than that of sexual offenses. In addition to the more liberalized definition of sexual assault, corroboration mandates were relaxed. However, reformers were less successful at abolishing the admissibility of marital immunity, prior sexual history evidence, and consent standards. The Rape Victim's Privacy Act, which was legislation designed to limit the extent to which evidence of the plaintiff's past sexual experience with people other than the defendant could be introduced in a sexual assault trial, was passed by Congress and signed by President Jimmy Carter in 1979. However, under many circumstances, the majority of states have allowed the defense to claim marital immunity, to ask about plaintiffs' prior sexual history, and to assert that consent was given (Sloan, 1992).

In 1974, one of the most liberal sexual assault laws to date was proposed in Michigan. This law had four main components: (1) an allowance for degrees of sexual assault that reflected an acknowledgment of the continuum of violence; (2) inadmissibility of sexual history evidence (except for evidence of prior sexual contact with the defendant and/or evidence of specific sexual activity that may show the source of semen, pregnancy, or disease); (3) repeal of resistance and consent standards; and (4) extension of the law to include sexual assault perpetrated by a female and homosexual sexual assault. However, even with these liberal elements, under some conditions (e.g., if the couple is married and living together), and in some circumstances, the sexual assault law may include a spousal exemption such that one spouse may not charge the other with rape (Sloan, 1992).

Overall, in the last 30 years, many sexual assault laws have reflected a more liberal, human rights approach to dealing with the legal issue of sexual aggression. Concurrently, the social conception of sexual aggression has been broadened. With the contemporary laws and social perceptions of sexual assault, female-perpetrated sexual aggression could be, theoretically, conceived. However, historically speaking, these laws have varied by state and have been in place for only a couple of decades. Even with all the advances that have taken place, current laws in approximately 12 of the states have not acknowledged female-perpetrated sexual coercion as a potential variation of sexual aggression (Sloan, 1992).

The broadened conception of sexual coercion reflected in changes in laws governing sexual assault are not generally reflected in the theories that guide researchers in developing research questions and designs nor in their interpretations of their data. We turn now to the theoretical assumptions underlying most research on sexual assault, including the assumption that men always have more power than do women.

## THEORIES, ASSUMPTIONS, AND THE SOCIAL CONSTRUCTION OF SEXUAL AGGRESSION IN RESEARCH

There have been three main, overlapping theoretical approaches proposed to explain sexual assault. These approaches have ranged from social psychological theories that focus on individual differences to sociocultural, feminist theories to more universal, evolutionary theories. All three operate on the assumption that men (*and not women*) are either socialized to be dominant and sexually aggressive or have a biological propensity to be so and that women (*and not men*) are socialized to be submissive or have a propensity to seek dominant, powerful males.

*Social psychological theorists* have generally relied on the discrepancy in personality traits of men who are sexually aggressive and women who are victimized. Specifically, researchers have described sexually aggressive men as exhibiting hypermasculine characteristics, such as strength, power, forcefulness, domination, and toughness (Mosher & Sirkin, 1984). In addition, in men who are sexually aggressive, these personality traits are likely to be combined with rape-supportive attitudes, generally aggressive or antisocial behavior, and a deviant sexual style (Burkhart & Fromuth, 1991). In contrast, researchers have suggested that women who adhere to a hyperfeminine personality style that is highly associated with traditional feminine gender roles might be vulnerable to sexual aggression. These hyperfeminine women are dependent and passive, viewing themselves as sexual objects and adhering to rape-supportive attitudes (Maybach & Gold, 1994).

Similarly, *feminist theorists* have taken some of these individual, social psychological models and extended them to reflect societal ways of thinking and behaving. Prevailing feminist explanations of sexual aggression have been based on the idea that sexual aggression or coercion is motivated by power and male dominance. That is, sexual aggression is primarily perpetrated by powerful men who attempt to maintain their power and dominance in society over relatively powerless and submissive women. Further, the power and dominance differentials between men and women are ingrained in society as a whole, such that sexual aggression by men toward women becomes an institutionalized and accepted way of interacting (Stock, 1991).

Other theorists have taken *evolutionarily derived ideas* and applied them to the realm of sexual aggression. One such evolutionary approach is based on the idea that during human evolutionary history there was enough selective pressure on males in favor of traits that solved the problem of procreation by forcing sex on a reluctant partner. Over many generations, the success of this force-oriented strategy produced psychological inclinations in men toward rape. Some evolutionary theorists have postulated that there were competing gender-specific pressures placed on individuals during the production of offspring. One key gender-specific behavioral observation related to the production of offspring is that women are more selective or discriminating in their choice of mates than are men. This gender discrepancy in mate selectivity has been attributed to greater parental investment by females than males (Trivers, 1972). Specifically, in human evolutionary history, women have had to make a larger investment in offspring than have men. Thus, women had more to lose than did men from a poor mate choice. Furthermore, because of this asymmetry in minimal investment in offspring, it was evolutionarily adaptive for women to have been more selective about mates and more interested in evaluating them and delaying copulation. For men, it was evolutionarily adaptive to copulate with many women to out reproduce men who preferred monogamy or who were less successful in obtaining sexual access to female partners. Given these gender-specific pressures and resultant behaviors, to have gained sexual access, men would have had to break through feminine barriers of hesitation and resistance. Thus, those men who used deceptive and coercive tactics, in addition to more honest advertisement, to gain greater sexual access would have had a reproductive advantage (Thornhill & Thornhill, 1991).

Overall, theorists using these three major approaches in attempting to explain sexual aggression have suggested that there are individual, societal, or even evolutionary forces that account for sexual aggression. However, the theories used to explain male perpetrator–female victim sexual coercion are the same stereotypes used to ignore the possibility of female perpetrator–male victim sexual coercion. Researchers who firmly adhere to these theoretical approaches to sexual aggression accept the assumption that the perpetrator of sexual aggression is a man and the victim is a woman. Thus, in the area of sexual aggression, theoretical assumptions may preclude researchers from exploring alternative types (female to male, female to female, or male to male) of sexual aggression.

Adherence to these theoretical approaches may combine with another very common tendency known as *confirmation bias* to limit our understanding of sexual assault. That is, laypersons and scientists alike tend to form hypotheses, seek confirmation of their hypotheses, and ignore disconfirming data. For example, in our roles as editor (Allgeier) and assistant editor (Lamping) of *The Journal of Sex Research,* we reviewed a manuscript in which the authors had provided men and women with a number of sexual scenarios that purportedly varied in the extent to which women were depicted in degrading situations. Overall, women had a significantly lower threshold for perceiving degradation in the sexual scenarios. However, an alert reviewer computed the correlation between men's and women's ratings and pointed out that they were highly correlated (.99). Had the authors been conducting intervention research aimed at sensitizing participants to degrading portrayals of women, they would have been delighted by the extent of agreement between men and women!

As will be described later, such confirmation bias is readily apparent in the work of Abbey (1982), Saal, Johnson, and Weber (1989), and others. Confirmation bias also appears in the work on the motives of perpetrators and victims in sexual coercion episodes.

## BELIEFS ABOUT ASSAILANTS' AND VICTIMS' MOTIVATIONS

With the growing power of the feminist movement in the 1970s, rape was reconceptualized as an act of violence and humiliation, compared to earlier views of rape as largely due to psychodynamic factors (e.g., Cohen, Garofalo, Boucher, & Seghorn, 1971) or "victim precipitation" (Amir, 1971). Feminist approaches have had some enduring, positive effects in bringing the seriousness of male-perpetrated sexual violations to the forefront as a societal and individual problem. However, sexual coercion research has also become deeply embedded within a political context of "violence," "victims," "survivors," "abusers," and "perpetrators," without adequate attention to men's (or women's) experiences beyond the realm of yes-or-no responses. In addition, exclusive adherence to feminist explanations of rape has been associated with the flat refusal of some researchers to consider the possibility that men may sometimes be the sexual targets of perpetrating women.

The current "politically correct" view of rapists as angry men motivated by desires to control, dominate, humiliate, and degrade hapless women dominates contemporary research on sexual assault. An article by Palmer (1988) titled "Twelve Reasons Why Rape Is Not Sexually Motivated: A Skeptical Examination" was one of the few exceptions to this portrayal of the rapist as an angry, power-driven man. Essentially, Palmer examined twelve arguments that rape is motivated by men's aggressive rather than sexual motives and concluded that all 12 arguments were "either logically unsound, based on inaccurate definitions, untestable, or inconsistent with the actual behavior of rapists" (p. 512). In the current climate, it is not surprising that Palmer's review has been largely ignored.

Omitted from Palmer's review was the fact that women can also be perpetrators. However, the first three studies documenting episodes of female perpetrators and male victims were published the same year as Palmer's review (Aizenman & Kelley, 1988; Muehlenhard & Cook, 1988; Struckman-Johnson, 1988), so he was presumably unaware of them at the time he wrote his article.

Groth's (1979) interviews with incarcerated men convicted of rape did support the portrayal of the rapist as an angry man who wanted to dominate and humiliate his victims, and presumably some rapists are motivated by such desires. However, an intriguing program of research by Freund and his colleagues (Freund & Blanchard, 1986; Freund, Scher, Racansky, Campbell, & Heasman, 1986) has led to the introduction of two new concepts relevant to the question of the motivation(s) of rapists. One of these is the *courtship disorders*. Working with men incarcerated for various sex offenses, including rape, Freund and his colleagues described a pattern in which many of these men proceeded directly to their sexual goal without bothering with the niceties of dating, kissing, petting, and so forth. Freund and associates essentially characterized these men as inept in their courtship behaviors. The other new concept is known as the *preferential rape pattern*. Specifically, men adhering to this pattern used only enough force to accomplish their sexual goals. If their victim appeared to be complying with the perpetrator's goal of having sex, the perpetrator ceased the use of force (Freund & Blanchard, 1986; Freund et al., 1986).

Other authors writing in this volume have studied and previously published articles about the apparent motives of women who coerce men to engage in unwanted sex (Anderson & Aymami, 1993; Craig, 1988).

To turn the whole question of motives for sexual aggression upside down, does the experimental induction of anger in men lead them to aggress toward a woman who has angered them? A considerable amount of research has demonstrated that men who are angered by women, shown violent pornography, and given the opportunity to behave aggressively by giving the woman negative evaluations or electric shocks do aggress to a greater extent than do men shown nonviolent pornography or not angered by a woman. In addition, men in the anger-induction, violent-pornography studies show increases in their acceptance of rape myths and violence toward women and in their self-reported likelihood to rape if they could be sure of not being caught (Check & Guloien, 1989; Demare, Briere, & Lips, 1988; Donnerstein & Berkowitz, 1981; Intons-Peterson, Roskos-Ewoldsen, Thomas, Shirley, & Blut, 1989; Malamuth & Check, 1981; Malamuth & Donnerstein, 1984). We know of no research employing the same paradigm with women volunteers who are shown violent pornography, angered by a male confederate, and subsequently given the opportunity to aggress against the man.

However, there is a preliminary finding that suggests that at least some of the earlier research demonstrating that angered men shown violent pornography and later allowed to aggress against a woman may have stemmed from demand characteristics in these lab studies. Fisher and Grenier (1994) used the same general paradigm with one major difference: Men were allowed to choose whether to shock the woman, give her verbal feedback, or simply leave the lab. Specifically, men were asked to write an essay that was subsequently evaluated negatively by a female confederate: "I was not impressed with the clarity or the content of this paper" (p. 33). In addition, the confederate delivered six brief electric shocks (using the Buss apparatus) to each man—a previous procedure with the men had established the level at which each found the shocks slightly uncomfortable or uncomfortable. Each man was then asked to participate in a supposedly separate pilot study by viewing violent pornography in which the woman victim was depicted as initially resisting sexual aggression but enjoying the rape by the end of the video (positive outcome).

After providing ratings of his arousal, each man returned to the room containing the shock-delivery apparatus. He was told to evaluate the memorization skills of the female confederate (supposedly another volunteer) who had previously shocked him. After the confederate (in another room) responded to each of 24 word pairs, the man was to inform the woman via microphone if her response was correct. The confederate gave correct responses to only one-third of the word pairs.

When the memory task was finished, each man was given one of three options: He could provide the woman with an overall evaluation of her performance by telling her over the intercom; he could evaluate her by delivering up to ten shocks (the greater the number of shocks, the more negative the evaluation); or he could skip the overall evaluation because he had already provided her with verbal feedback following each word pair. If he chose the last alternative, he could move directly to debriefing. That alternative had not been provided in early studies of men's responses to being angered and shown violent pornography, but when given it, 64% of the men chose to be debriefed without delivering an overall evaluation. The 21% of the men who chose to speak with the woman did so in a pleasant and nonaggressive fashion. The men who chose to deliver shock (14%) *"had verbalized considerable eagerness to use the Buss apparatus when they were first introduced to it and well before they had viewed the violent stimulus"* (p. 35, emphasis in original) or had been provoked by the confederate. Overall, 86% of the men showed no physically aggressive behavior.

Our use of percentages in reporting Fisher and Grenier's findings may be somewhat misleading. One of the limitations of the study is that only 14 men participated in it. However, the authors noted: "Because the fundamental experimental question—whether violent pornography reliably causes antiwoman aggression in a laboratory setting that possesses ecologically representative options—had been answered clearly, there was no point in gratuitously exposing additional subjects to additional verbal provocation, electric shock, violent pornography, and other such procedures" (p. 35).

Clearly, this study should be replicated by independent researchers with a larger sample of men *and women*. Would women be even less likely to aggress when angered by a male confederate and shown violent pornography involving a female perpetrator and a male victim? Although we view this study as providing very preliminary evidence that the majority of men are likely just to walk away when provoked by a woman, shown violent pornography, and given the alternative of aggressing against the woman, it certainly does not support the hypothesis that men who are angered are invariably going to take their anger out on a woman by aggressing against her.

Again, note the underlying assumption pervading almost all research in this area: It is men who aggress and women who are victimized. This same built-in bias pervades other experimental and survey studies. That is, until 1988, with the publication of the three studies noted earlier, only men were asked about their own aggressive behavior (but not about being victims of sexual aggression) and only women were asked about victimization (but not about their sexual coercion of men).

## THE FRAMING OF RESEARCH QUESTIONS

The problem of misinterpretation of the neutral point or midpoint of measurement scales (and confirmation bias, which we defined earlier) also plagues research purportedly aimed at explaining sexual assault. More than a decade ago, Abbey (1982) published an article that continues to be widely cited in research articles and in texts in the social sciences. She posed a question in her title: "Sex Differences in Attributions for Friendly Behavior: Do Males Misperceive Females' Friendliness?" Essentially, she assigned college men and women volunteers to one of two conditions. They were either to engage in a conversation with a member of the other gender while being observed through one-way glass or to be observers of the conversants. After observing the dyads engage in the 5-minute conversation about their experiences that year at college, observers were asked to rate the man and woman regarding how each was "trying to behave." To measure sexual intent, "the key trait terms were the adjectives *flirtatious, seductive,* and *promiscuous.* These terms were selected because they were thought to measure the construct 'sexuality' " (p. 833). Abbey imbedded these three terms in a variety of trait terms, using 7-point response formats. No gender differences emerged in volunteers' ratings of the women actors' friendliness, and the ratings were high on the 7-point scale (mean for women = 6.0; for men, 5.7).

Regarding her measures of sexual intent, Abbey (1982) reported that: "as predicted, male subjects rated the female actor as being significantly *more promiscuous* than female subjects did ($p < .01$). Similarly, there was a marginal effect for males to rate the female actor as being *more seductive* than did females ($p < .09$). However, there were no sex differences in subjects' ratings of the female's flirtatiousness" (pp. 833–834, emphasis added). Note that promiscuity, seductiveness, and flirtatiousness were rated on 7-point scales, with 1 indicating the *absence* of the quality and 7 indicating its *presence.* Inspection of the means actually suggests that men and women alike gave low ratings on all three characteristics. In judging the women actors, men versus women observers gave mean ratings of the women's promiscuity of 2.2 versus 1.7, of seductiveness, 2.3 versus 1.9, and of flirtatiousness, 2.9 versus 2.8. Note that only one rating—promiscuous (or, more accurately taking into account the issue of the neutral point, *not* promiscuous)—reached statistical significance. Even so, the difference between 2.2 versus 1.7, only half of one scale point, raises questions about effect size. Specifically, although a significant difference was found on this one variable, the meaningfulness of the difference—at the not-promiscuous end of the scale—is small. That is, neither men nor women rated the stimulus as promiscuous, and women were slightly less likely to do so.

Now, let's examine Abbey's abstract. Essentially, her interpretation of the answer to her question "Do Males Misperceive Females' Friendliness?" was "yes."

This investigation tested the hypothesis that friendliness from a member of the opposite sex might be misperceived as a sign of sexual interest. Previous research in the area of acquaintance and date rape suggests that males frequently misunderstand females' intentions. A laboratory experiment was conducted in which a male and a female participated in a 5-minute conversation while a hidden male and female observed this interaction. The results indicate that there were sex differences in subjects' ratings of the actors. Male actors and observers rated the female actor as being more promiscuous and seductive than female actors and observers rated her. Males were also more sexually attracted to the opposite-sex actor than females were. Furthermore, males also rated the male actor in a more sexualized fashion than females did. These results were interpreted as indicating that men are more likely to perceive the world in sexual terms and to make sexual judgments than women are. Males do seem to perceive friendliness from females as seduction, but this appears to be merely one manifestation of a broader male sexual orientation. (p. 830)

The dangers of data in our abstracts being misinterpreted are exacerbated by the hectic schedule under which popular-press writers and textbook authors operate. We could give a litany of how Abbey's data have been reported in secondary sources. Check the textbooks on your shelves. We will give just one example, because it occurred in the third edition of a social psychology text we have used by David Myers (1993). Here is his text description:

Indeed, our conclusions about why people act as they do are profoundly important. They determine our reactions to people and our decisions regarding them. For example, Antonia Abbey (1987) and her colleagues have repeatedly found that men are more likely than women to attribute a woman's friendliness to sexual interest. This misreading of warmth as a sexual come-on (an example of a "misattribution") can lead to inappropriate behavior and helps explain the greater sexual assertiveness exhibited by men across the world (Kenrick & Trost, 1987). Such misattributions can also contribute both to date rape and to the greater tendency of men in various cultures, from Boston to Bombay, to justify rape by blaming the victim's behavior (Kanekar & Nazareth, 1988; Muehlenhard, 1988; Shotland, 1989). (Myers, 1993, p. 75)

One of us (Allgeier) knows Dave Myers and wrote him about his rendering of Abbey's findings. Myers wrote back a very sweet letter, essentially saying, "Oh, you are right, and I've made it worse in the fourth edition" (Myers, personal communication, ca. 1994), which was already in press. Actually, all he did in his fourth edition was to add sexual harassment to the list of behaviors experienced by women as a function of men's "misattributions," citing research by another group in which the means were much closer to the "absence" than to the "presence" end of sexual intent.

It is easy to sound holier-than-thou on the issue of interpreting ratings. Last year, I (Allgeier) decided to reexamine my own dissertation, completed in 1976. The relevant study was published in the *Journal of Consulting and Clinical Psychology* (Allgeier & Fogel, 1978). I manipulated gender role behavior in the context of a sexual interaction. Specifically, I showed slides of the same couple engaged in coitus in either the man-above or woman-above position. Students rated the man and woman in the slides along a number of dimensions and also completed a measure of gender role identification. I expected that traditional students, compared to androgynous students, would rate both the man and the woman in the woman-above position more negatively than they would rate the couple in the man-above position. Gender role identification was unrelated to ratings of the man and woman in the slides, but student gender was a strong predictor. Gender differences emerged on six of the nine ratings of the woman in the slides and on four of the nine ratings of the man in the slides. For example, on a scale ranging from "dirty" (1) to "clean" (7), mean ratings given by the women to the woman in the man-above versus woman-above condition were 6.17 versus 5.38, respectively ($p < .01$). Similarly, in ratings on the dimension from "immoral" to "moral," the means by women for women in the man-above versus women-above condition were 5.92 versus 4.88, respectively ($p < .005$). Similar judgments were made about the man in the man-above versus woman-above conditions. But here's what I wrote about the results displayed in the relevant table presented in my dissertation:

> Internal comparisons revealed that females consistently rated the couple in the woman-above position more negatively that they did the couple in the man-above position. Specifically, the woman was rated as dirtier, less respectable, less moral, less good, less desirable as a wife, and less desirable as a mother when she was on top than when she was beneath the man during intercourse. Females also rated the man as dirtier, less respectable, less moral, and less masculine when he was in the woman-above

position than when he was in the man-above position. (Allgeier, 1976, p. 21)

Not one of those statements is accurate; in fact, women rated the woman in the man-above position as cleaner, more respectable, more moral, and so forth. With a neutral point of 4, the woman in neither set of slides was rated as dirty, unrespectable, immoral, and so forth. In retrospect, I would not recommend acceptance of my own study as I then wrote it, but my doctoral committee did, and the *Journal of Consulting and Clinical Psychology* did.

You may think that this issue is trivial, and with respect to my own study, I don't think that my error in interpreting my findings has made much of an impact. The point is that we can be biased by the way we think about our research questions into seeking confirmation of our beliefs and hypotheses. We should also be alert to alternative interpretations and conduct analyses to see if they could also be supported.

## MEASURING SEXUAL COERCION

We turn now to the measurement of unwanted sex. What we discuss next is controversial and is one instance of what has been perceived by some people as undermining the "feminist agenda" regarding sexual coercion and rape. However, we need as much valid information as possible if we are to develop intervention strategies to reduce the prevalence of sexual coercion.

In 1990, an advertisement from the Rape Treatment Center (RTC) of Santa Monica Hospital had bold headlines and was widely distributed to colleges:

> Think of the six women
> closest to you.
> Now guess
> which one will be raped
> this year.

This headline was followed by text claiming that one out of six college women would be sexually assaulted that year. Advice was provided regarding safety precautions. When interviewed, personnel at the RTC acknowledged that its statistic was too high (Schoenberg & Roe, 1993). Included in the statistic were behaviors ranging from unwanted touching to rape. Where did the statistic come from? It was based on a 1987 survey conducted by psychologist Mary Koss and sponsored by *Ms.* magazine. In this mammoth study, students at 32 colleges were given the Sexual Experiences Survey (SES), a 12-item measure of unwanted sexual behaviors (Koss, Gidycz, & Wisniewski, 1987). The SES, originally designed by Koss and Oros (1982), and subsequent modifications of it is the most widely used measure of sexual coercion (Porter & Critelli, 1992). Consistent with our earlier discussion of the bias that is introduced by assuming that men are always the perpetrators and women are always the victims, the version administered to men asked about their coercive behavior. The version administered to women inquires about their victimization experiences.

Ross and Allgeier (1996) were interested in men's interpretation of a third of the SES items (Koss & Oros, 1982). We obtained a release from the U.S. government that permitted the questioning of volunteers without having to report their responses or identity to authorities and told the men about that release. The 102 men first responded to the SES. Each man was then interviewed about his interpretations of the four items that appeared to be ambiguously worded (2, 3, 5, and 6) and which pilot data had indicated that some respondents found vague. Each item begins with the phrase "Have you ever . . . ?" Item 2 continues, "had a woman misinterpret the level of sexual intimacy you desired?" Item 3 says "been in a sexual situation where you became so sexually aroused that you could not stop yourself even though the woman did not want to?" Item 5 continues, "had sexual intercourse with a woman when she didn't really want to because she felt pressured by your continual arguments?" Item 6 states "obtained intercourse by saying things you really didn't mean?"

Almost all the men (93%) reported that they had experienced consensual vaginal intercourse and/or oral sex with a woman. In presenting the categories of interpretation for the four items hypothesized to be ambiguous, Ross and Allgeier (1996) distilled the intended meanings of each item into a "prototypic" interpretation. Space doesn't permit a detailed description of varying interpretations of the meaning of all four items, but we will review the findings for Item 3. Overall, 60% of the men interpreted the meaning of Item 3 (which has no real behavioral referent) as asking whether they specifically had *vaginal penetration* with a woman because of loss of control over their sex drive, an interpretation presumably consistent with the interpretations of researchers using the SES for classifying men into rapist and nonrapist groups.

However, 40% of the men had different interpretations of this item. Some of these men interpreted the item as referring to doing *anything sexual* with a woman when she did not desire it. These men saw the item as asking whether they had any type of sexual contact with a woman against her wishes, such as touching or kissing. Overall, 33.3% of the entire sample held this interpretation, and all responded "no" to the item.

A small group of men whose interpretations didn't fit that category were identified. Of these seven men, two men who responded "no" interpreted the item as asking whether they had become sexually aroused "visually," such as might happen when watching a woman dance. Other interpretations included situations during which the man eventually *did stop,* although he felt "out of control" for a brief period. The behavior he was referring to was petting, and *intercourse never occurred* during the event in question. He reported that there was no indication from the woman that he was coercive. A second man reported that he eventually *did stop* during a sexual encounter but that he felt "out of control" for a brief period. He was referring to kissing a woman and touching her breasts over her sweater, and *intercourse never occurred.* He reported that the woman gave no indication that he was coercive. A third man stated that he was referring to a situation during which he did stop attempts to pet, but he could not stop himself from continuing to *ask her to have intercourse* when she refused. There was no indication that he behaved coercively; rather, he seemed to believe that his asking her to have intercourse made it appropriate for him to respond "yes" to the item. He interpreted "could not stop . . . " as referring to "stopping myself from asking her" to have intercourse. A fourth man recalled a situation during which he was receiving oral sex and he ejaculated when the woman wanted him to delay ejaculation. He therefore responded "yes" because he interpreted the "could not stop" phrase as meaning ejaculating. The fifth man recalled a situation during which he *could not stop kissing* (consensual kissing) after a woman refused to have intercourse. He therefore interpreted the item as asking whether he ever continued to feel aroused to the degree that he wanted to continue consensual "foreplay" after having advances rejected. Presumably, many men (and women) have had these kinds of experiences, but should they be classified as rapists?

The SES and altered versions have been used in three major ways. First, some researchers examine SES responses and categorize men into various groups based on the perceived level of sexual coercion that men admit to by their distribution of "yes" responses. For example, a man responding "yes" to SES item 10 ("Have you ever had sexual intercourse with a women when she didn't want to because you threatened to use physical force [twisting her arm, holding her down, etc.] if she didn't cooperate?") is typically assigned the label of "rapist." In contrast, a man responding "yes" to only a less "serious" item such as item 5 ("Have you ever had sexual intercourse with a woman when she didn't really want to because she felt pressured by your continual arguments?") may be called "coercive" (e.g., Koss, Leonard, Beezley, & Oros, 1985; Lisak & Roth, 1988). Second, others have chosen only one item, such as item 3 (Craig, 1988), and dichotomized men into "coercive" versus "noncoercive" groups according to whether a man responded "yes" or "no" to the item. Third, others have used the SES or an alteration and computed coercion "scores," whereby a "yes" response to any item other than to item 1 ("Have you ever had sexual intercourse with a woman when you both wanted to?") earns a man a "point" toward a total index of his "coerciveness" (e.g., Malamuth, 1986; Peterson & Franzese, 1987). The results of Ross and Allgeier's (1996) study of men's interpretations of the items have implications for these major uses of the SES. Specifically, men may be potentially categorized inaccurately as to their level of sexual "coerciveness."

For example, item 3 ("could not stop") was dropped from at least one researcher's analyses because he perceived it as too "vague" (e.g., Malamuth, 1986). Ironically, item 3 continues to be used in the assessment of coercive sexual behavior. In fact, that one item alone was used as the basis for the assignment of men to "coercive" ("yes" responses) and "noncoercive" ("no" responses) groups (Craig, 1993). In her published report of the research, Craig wrote "[have sexual intercourse]" in brackets after the item (p. 420). When asked if the bracketed material had also been on the measures to which her volunteers responded, she candidly acknowledged that it was not. Ross and Allgeier's (1996) data provided statistical evidence that "yes" responses on item 3 were significantly more likely among men who reported interpretations not related to a coercive incident. Specifically, of the six "yes" responders in their sample, five out of six men interpreted the item as referring to a situation perceived to be devoid of coercion.

For the four items assessed by Ross and Allgeier (1996), it is clear that "yes" responses did not necessarily denote coercive behavior. Similarly, responses of "no" did not necessarily represent a *lack* of coercive behavior on the part of a given man. Item interpretations may lead to inaccurate labeling of men's behavior either in the direction of overestimating or underestimating a man's level of coerciveness. Based on Ross and Allgeier's findings, it appears that researchers must evaluate interpretations in assessing both "yes" and "no" responses to SES items.

Although a few studies have recently been published that measure sexually coercive behavior by either men or women, the prevailing common assumption that, in coercive contacts, men are always the perpetrators and women are always the victims will remain unchallenged until our research designs and measures ask about the roles people have in sexually coercive episodes, regardless of their gender. In that regard, researchers should administer measures of sexual coercion to women to obtain their interpretation of the questions and measures of being victimized to men to obtain their interpretations.

## RESEARCHERS' INTERPRETATIONS IN SEXUAL COERCION RESEARCH

Earlier, we discussed researchers' and writers' interpretations (and misinterpretations) of their own and others' data. We addressed in several sections the problem of confirmation bias and the neutral point on scales. Much of the research using the SES demonstrates these problems.

Hull and Burke (1991) referred to any "yes" response on the original SES as an "abusive act." The use of such language has served to "smooth" research outcomes and ignore item interpretations and behavioral referents that critically define the nature of a given sexual interaction.

Attempts have been made to develop a "unified" theory of

sexual aggression capable of accounting for both the similarities and differences among all sexually aggressive males by identifying key motivational factors in men's (but not women's) coercive behavior (e.g., Hall, 1990; Hall & Hirschman, 1991; Knight & Prentky, 1990; Malamuth, 1986; Malamuth, Sockloskie, Koss, & Tanaka, 1991; Prentky & Knight, 1991; Shotland, 1989). Following the assumptions underlying this model has led researchers such as Malamuth et al. (1991) to approach all SES items as reflecting an underlying level of "aggression" toward women, whether it be verbal or physical attempts to gain sexual access.

If a man interprets an SES item as asking if exaggerated flattery has been used on a woman, then his response may be grouped with other "yes" responses and collectively referred to as "coercive" in the current climate of methodology and language in the United States. On the basis of their data, Ross and Allgeier (1996) asserted that it is inaccurate to equate flattery, exaggerated emotional investment, and talking a person into a sexual interaction with forcibly removing a person's ability to consent. Doing so appears to assume an unreasonable definition of what "consent" represents. A person who is "sweet-talked" home from a bar cannot be seen as "victimized" in the same way as a person whose ability to consent has been taken by physical force.

In addition to its use with men, the SES has historically been used to classify women as to levels of "victimization." For example, an item worded for women states: "Have you had sexual intercourse when you didn't want to because a man gave you alcohol or drugs?" A woman's affirmative response to this item in the Koss et al. (1987) study resulted in her being categorized as having been "raped."

There are two important issues here. First, unless the female is a child, or the man has forced her to drink or take drugs or has slipped her a "mickey" or "roofie," she is presumably free to choose the extent to which she imbibes intoxicants. As Gilbert (1993) observed, the meaning of having sex "because" a man gave you drugs is unclear. An affirmative response says nothing about duress, intoxication, the woman's judgment or control, or whether a man intentionally got a woman drunk for the purpose of reducing her resistance to having sex with him. He also suggested that the item might be interpreted to mean that a woman traded sex for drugs or that a small level of alcohol lowered a woman's inhibitions and she consented to an act she later regretted. It is also possible that the man in the interaction subsequently regretted having had sex (Roiphe, 1993).

Second, we know of no published research in which men are asked, "Have you had sexual intercourse when you didn't want to because a woman gave you alcohol or drugs?" with men's affirmative answers yielding the classification of the man as having been "raped." The editors of this book have both reported on women getting men drunk or drugged to have sex with them. Neither of these researchers chose to classify this behavior as "rape" (Anderson, 1995; Struckman-Johnson & Struckman-Johnson, 1994).

Third, we will briefly mention a different aspect of the notion of unwanted sex. Does all unwanted sex involve coercion by a man (or woman) of a woman (or man)? That is, does a "yes" answer to a "when you didn't want to" question always imply that the other person forced you to engage in sexual interaction? Or is it possible that many of us experience unwanted *consensual* sex from time to time? Most of us who have been in an ongoing relationship for an extended period of time will probably recognize that there are instances in which our partner desires sex with us when we are not feeling sexual desire. However, we may comply with our partner's interest in getting together sexually and may not indicate our relative disinclination for sex at that particular time. Some of us occasionally feign interest in sexual activity when it is apparent that our partner wants to get together, and in many cases our initially lukewarm feelings heat up during the interaction, even though, given our feelings at the outset, we would have preferred to do something else. Several studies have documented the existence of unwanted ("when you didn't want to") consensual sex (Sprecher, Hatfield, Cortese, Potapova, & Levitskaya, 1994; O'Sullivan & Allgeier, 1998). These studies may suggest that researchers who classify people as victims or rapists on the basis of questions about unwanted sex may have confounded the prevalence of unwanted nonconsensual sexual contacts with unwanted, but consensual, sexual interactions. It should be obvious at this point that we believe that our measures of coercive sex need to be phrased such that it is abundantly clear that the unwanted sex was actually coerced by the "perpetrator" from the recipient against his or her will.

## CONCLUSIONS AND RECOMMENDATIONS
## FOR FUTURE RESEARCH

To summarize this voyage along the dimensions from consensual to coercive sex, we think that it is critical that we researchers acknowledge our values. We need to guard against questions and measures, designs, and analyses that can only confirm, but not disconfirm, our hypotheses.

One constructive move in this direction is to provide men and women with measures in which they can report experiences with forced sex—in the roles of both perpetrating coercion *and* being the recipient of coercion—and to ask them the approximate dates of these experiences. A frequently presented public awareness message on television several years ago asserted that men incarcerated for sexual offenses had themselves been abused earlier when they were children. However, many of us who experienced psychological and sexual abuse when we were children did not become adults who emotionally or sexually abuse or assault others. We have very little information available to allow us to determine the extent of the correlation between past experiences of being abused and subsequent abuse or assault of nonconsenting "partners."

We also need to attend to the neutral-point (or midpoint) issue in evaluating research outcomes. Unfortunately, because of confirmation bias in which differences arise between the actual data obtained by researchers and their interpretations of such, we can be misled if we attend only to researchers' own interpretations of their findings.

Further, our attempts to measure coercive sex should include items containing behavioral referents that indicate what we actually mean by unwanted sex. That is, we should ask respondents who indicate having experienced coerced sex (as "giver" or "receiver") how they knew that the sexual episode was unwanted. Bart (1981) conducted a very instructive study of women who had both experienced attempted rapes and been successful in avoiding rapes. Those episodes in which women gave a single message that they did not want to engage in sexual activity were more likely to result in rape. In contrast, in other coercion experiences in which the same women used multiple messages to convey their disinclination to have sex, the women were more successful in avoiding coerced sex. Her study needs to be replicated with men who have experienced attempted sexual coercion by women.

Finally, although we have not previously mentioned it in this chapter, there is the issue of reconstructing past events. That is, one may construe events with a current sexual partner differently from how one construes interactions with past partners. It is common for young people (e.g., college students) to describe their current relationships as involving love but to describe their past relationships as just "puppy love." We are not sure what "puppy love" is in the minds of people in their late adolescence. For that matter, we also do not know why a current relationship is perceived as involving "real love." Thus, it might be helpful to ask respondents how they defined past events at the time that they occurred versus how they now perceive those past events. This has been done with research on sexual harassment in academic settings, and students report more negative evaluations of their interactions with instructors currently than they did at the time that the episode took place (Allgeier, Travis, Zeller, & Royster, 1990).

Unfortunately, forced sexual contacts are a reality and seem to have been so for all recorded history. However, to understand this phenomenon and to attempt to reduce its frequency, we need to have as much accurate data as possible. We hope that our review of the various forms of distortion in research in this area will help to increase the quality of the research that we conduct. Only by trying to provide accurate reporting of the phenomenon of sexual coercion will we be able to obtain useful data that can be employed to try to reduce the prevalence of the use of coercion by men and women to force others to engage in unwanted sexual contacts.

## REFERENCES

Abbey, A. (1982). Sex differences in attributions for friendly behavior. Do males misperceive females' friendliness? *Journal of Personality and Social Psychology, 42,* 830–838.

Abbey, A. (1987). Misperceptions of friendly behavior as sexual interest: A survey of naturally occurring incidents. *Psychology of Women Quarterly, 11,* 173–194.

Aizenman, M., & Kelley, G. (1988). The incidence of violence and acquaintance rape in dating relationships among college men and women. *Journal of College Student Development, 29,* 305–311.

Allgeier, E. R. (1976). *The influence of sex roles on heterosexual attitudes and behavior.* Unpublished doctoral dissertation, Purdue University.

Allgeier, E. R., & Fogel, A. (1978). Coital positions and sex roles: Responses to cross-sex behavior in bed. *Journal of Consulting and Clinical Psychology, 46,* 588–589.

Allgeier, E., Travis, S., Zeller, R., & Royster, B. (1990, March). *Constructions of consensual versus coercive sex: A survey of student–instructor sexual contacts.* Paper presented at the Western Region meeting of the Society for the Scientific Study of Sex, San Francisco.

Amir, M. (1971). *Patterns in forcible rape.* Chicago: University of Chicago Press.

Anderson, P. (1995, November). Women's motives for heterosexual initiation and aggression. In C. Muehlenhard (Chair), *Sexual coercion of men by women: Implications for the role of gender and the role of politics in sexual science.* Symposium presented at the annual meeting of The Society for the Scientific Study of Sex, San Francisco, CA.

Anderson, P., & Aymami, R. (1993). Reports of female initiation of sexual contact: Male and female differences. *Archives of Sexual Behavior, 22*(4), 335–343.

Bart, P. (1981). A study of women who both were raped and avoided rape. *Journal of Sexual Issues, 37*(4), 123–137.

Black, H. (1968). *Black's law dictionary.* St. Paul, MN: West.

Burkhart, B., & Fromuth, M. (1991). Individual psychological and social psychological understandings of sexual coercion. In E. Grauerholz & M. A. Koralewski (Eds.), *Sexual coercion: A sourcebook on its nature, causes, and prevention* (pp. 75–89). Lexington, MA: Lexington Books.

Check, J., & Guloien, T. (1989). Reported proclivity for coercive sex following repeated exposure to sexually violent pornography, nonviolent dehumanizing pornography, and erotica. In D. Zillmann & J. Bryant (Eds.), *Pornography: Research advances and policy considerations* (pp. 159–184). Hillsdale, NJ: Erlbaum.

Cohen, M., Garofalo, R., Boucher, R., & Seghorn, T. (1971). The psychology of rapists. *Seminars in Psychiatry, 3,* 307–327.

Craig, M. (1988). The sexually coercive college female: An investigation of attitudinal and affective characteristics. In C. Muehlenhard (Chair), *Sexually coerced men and sexually coercive women.* Symposium presented at the annual meeting of the Society for The Scientific Study of Sex, San Francisco.

Craig, M. (1993). The effects of selective evaluation on the perception of female cues in sexually coercive and noncoercive males. *Archives of Sexual Behavior, 22,* 415–433.

Demare, D., Briere, J., & Lips, H. (1988). Violent pornography and self-reported likelihood of sexual aggression. *Journal of Research in Personality, 22,* 140–155.

Dixon, J. (1991). Feminist reforms of sexual coercion laws. In E. Grauerholz

& M. A. Koralewski (Eds.), *Sexual coercion: A sourcebook on its nature, causes, and prevention* (pp. 161–171). Lexington, MA: Lexington Books.

Donnerstein, E., & Berkowitz, L. (1981). Victim reactions in aggressive erotic films as a factor in violence against women. *Journal of Personality and Social Psychology, 41,* 710–724.

Fisher, W., & Grenier, G. (1994). Violent pornography, antiwoman thoughts, and antiwoman acts: In search of reliable effects. *Journal of Sex Research, 31,* 23–38.

Freund, K., & Blanchard, R. (1986). The concept of courtship disorder. *Journal of Sex and Marital Therapy, 12,* 79–92.

Freund, K., Scher, H., Racansky, I. G., Campbell, K., & Heasman, J. (1986). Males disposed to rape. *Archives of Sexual Behavior, 15,* 23–35.

Gilbert, N. (1993). Realities and mythologies of rape. In *Annual editions: Human sexuality* (1993/94) (pp. 211–217). Guilford, CT: Dushkin.

Groth, A. (1979). *Men who rape: The psychology of the offender.* New York: Plenum Press.

Hall, G.(1990). Prediction of sexual aggression. *Clinical Psychology Review, 10,* 229–246.

Hall, G., & Hirschman, R. (1991). Toward a theory of sexual aggression: A quadripartite model. *Journal of Consulting and Clinical Psychology, 59,* 662–669.

Hull, D., & Burke, J. (1991). The religious right, attitudes toward women, and tolerance for sexual abuse. *Journal of Offender Rehabilitation, 17*(1), 1–12.

Intons-Peterson, M., Roskos-Ewoldsen, B., Thomas, L., Shirley, M., & Blut, D. (1989). Will educational materials reduce negative effects of exposure to sexual violence? *Journal of Social and Clinical Psychology, 8,* 256–275.

Kanekar, S., & Nazareth, A. (1988). Attributed rape victim's fault as a function of her attractiveness, physical hurt, and emotional disturbance. *Social Behavior, 3,* 37–40.

Kenrick, D., & Trost, M. (1987). A biosocial theory of heterosexual relationships. In K. Kelly (Ed.), *Females, males, and sexuality* (pp. 59–100). Albany, NY: State University of New York Press.

Knight, R., & Prentky, R. (1990). Classifying sexual offenders: The development and corroboration of taxonomic models. In W. L. Marshall, D. R. Laws, & H. E. Barbaree (Eds.), *Handbook of sexual assault: Issues, theories, and treatment of the offender* (pp. 23–52). New York: Plenum Press.

Koss, M., Gidycz, C., & Wisniewski, N. (1987). The scope of rape: Incidence and prevalence of sexual aggression and victimization in a national sample of higher education students. *Journal of Consulting and Clinical Psychology, 55,* 162–170.

Koss, M., Leonard, K., Beezley, D., & Oros, C. (1985). Nonstranger sexual aggression: A discriminant analysis of the psychological characteristics of undetected offenders. *Sex Roles, 12,* 981–992.

Koss, M., & Oros, C. (1982). Sexual Experiences Survey: A research instrument investigating sexual aggression and victimization. *Journal of Consulting and Clinical Psychology, 50,* 455–457.

Lisak, D., & Roth, S. (1988). Motivational factors in nonincarcerated sexually aggressive men. *Journal of Personality and Social Psychology, 55,* 795–802.

Malamuth, N. (1986). Predictors of naturalistic sexual aggression. *Journal of Personality and Social Psychology, 50,* 953–962.

Malamuth, N., & Check, J. (1981). The effects of mass media exposure on acceptance of violence against women: A field experiment. *Journal of Research in Personality, 15,* 436–446.

Malamuth, N., & Donnerstein, E. (Eds.). (1984). *Pornography and sexual aggression.* Orlando, FL: Academic Press.

Malamuth, N., Sockloskie, R., Koss, M., & Tanaka, J. (1991). Characteristics of aggressors against women: Testing a model using a national sample of college students. *Journal of Consulting and Clinical Psychology, 59,* 670–681.

Maybach, K., & Gold, S. (1994). Hyperfemininity and attraction to macho and non-macho men. *Journal of Sex Research, 31,* 91–98.

Mosher, D., & Sirkin, M. (1984). Measuring a macho personality constellation. *Journal of Research in Personality, 18,* 150–163.

Muehlenhard, C. (1988a). Misinterpreting dating behaviors and the risk of date rape. *Journal of Social and Clinical Psychology, 6,* 20–37.

Muehlenhard, C., & Cook, S. (1988). Men's self-reports of unwanted sexual activity. *Journal of Sex Research, 24,* 58–72.

Myers, D. (1993). *Social psychology* (3rd ed.). New York: McGraw-Hill.

O'Sullivan, L., & Allgeier, E. (1998). Feigning sexual interest: Consenting to unwanted sexual activity in heterosexual dating relationships. *Journal of Sex Resesarch, 35*(3).

Palmer, C. (1988). Twelve reasons why rape is not sexually motivated: A skeptical examination. *Journal of Sex Research, 25,* 512–530.

Peterson, S., & Franzese, B. (1987). Correlates of college men's sexual abuse of women. *Journal of College Student Personnel, 28,* 223–228.

Porter, J., & Critelli, J. (1992). Measurement of sexual aggression in college men: A methodological analysis. *Archives of Sexual Behavior, 21,* 525–542.

Prentky, R., & Knight, R. (1991). Identifying critical dimensions for discriminating among rapists. *Journal of Consulting and Clinical Psychology, 59,* 643–661.

Reiss, I. (1993). The future of sex research and the meaning of science. *Journal of Sex Research, 30,* 3–11.

Roiphe, K. (1993). *The morning after: Sex, fear, and feminism on campus.* Boston: Little, Brown.

Ross, R., & Allgeier, E. (1996). Behind the pencil/paper measurement of sexual coercion: Interview-based clarification of men's interpretations of Sexual Experience Survey items. *Journal of Applied Social Psychology, 26,* 1587–1616.

Saal, F., Johnson, C., & Weber, N. (1989). Friendly or sexy? It may depend on whom you ask. *Psychology of Women Quarterly, 13,* 263–276.

Schoenberg, N., & Roe, S. (1993, November 17). Erroneous statistic on rape stands uncorrected. *Toledo Blade,* pp. 1, 7.

Shotland, R. (1989). A model of the causes of date rape in developing and close relationships. In C. Hendrick (Ed.), *Review of personality and social psychology* (Vol. 10). Beverly Hills, CA: Sage.

Sloan, I. (1992). *Rape.* Dobbs Ferry, NY: Oceana.

Sprecher, S., Hatfield, E., Cortese, A., Potapova, E., & Levitskaya, A. (1994). Token resistance to sexual intercourse and consent to un-wanted sexual intercourse: College students' dating experiences in three countries. *Journal of Sex Research, 31,* 125–132.

Stock, W. (1991). Feminist explanations: Male power, hostility, and sexual coercion. In E. Grauerholz & M. A. Koralewski (Eds.), *Sexual coercion: A sourcebook on its nature, causes, and prevention* (pp. 62–73). Lexington, MA: Lexington Books.

Struckman-Johnson, C. (1988). Forced sex on dates: It happens to men, too. *Journal of Sex Research, 24,* 234–241.

Struckman-Johnson, C., & Struckman-Johnson, D. (1994). Men pressured and forced into sexual experience. *Archives of Sexual Behavior, 23*(1), 93–114.

Thornhill, R., & Thornhill, N. (1992). The evolutionary psychology of men's coercive sexuality. *Behavioral and Brain Sciences, 15,* 363–375.

Trivers, R. (1972). Parental investment and sexual selection. In B. Campbell (Ed.), *Sexual selection and the descent of man* (pp. 136–179). Chicago: Aldine.

# II

## TRAITS AND MOTIVES
## OF SEXUALLY
## AGGRESSIVE WOMEN

There is much to learn about the characteristics and motives of sexually aggressive women. Peter B. Anderson and Mary E. Craig Shea, authors of Chapters 4 and 5, are among the few researchers to date who have studied women who admit to sexually aggressive behavior. Anderson reviews results of his dissertation and his continued work on the relationship among past sexual abuse, adversarial beliefs, and sexually aggressive behavior in women. He presents his findings on women's self-reports of motives for heterosexual aggression and the strategies used to initiate sex with men, including several that could be considered coercive or aggressive. Shea examines motives of college women who used verbal coercion to have sex with men. Like Anderson, Shea presents evidence that sexually aggressive women can be distinguished by their social histories and belief systems.

In Chapter 6, Lee Ellis, author of several books on theories of rape, proposes a "biosocial" explanation for women's sexual aggression. Extending his previous work on evolutionary perspectives on male sexual coercion, Ellis suggests that a proportion of women coerce men into sex because of their biological drives for sex and dominance. Ellis combines the results of numerous studies to test the proposition that women are most likely to use pressure or psychological tactics rather than physical force to coerce men into sex.

# 4

# Women's Motives for Sexual Initiation and Aggression

## PETER B. ANDERSON

In 1927, Bronislaw Malinowski reported to the scientific community on several aspects of women's sexual aggression among tribal cultures in the Trobriand Islands. These aggressive acts included group attacks on men from other tribes, culminating in forced sexual intercourse. The men suffering from these onslaughts were ridiculed and humiliated, as well as physically beaten and abused by their attackers (Malinowski, 1927). It is possible that these reports were only legends that served some unknown purpose for the tribes involved, but it is certain that more recent reports of women's sexual aggression in the United States reflect real-life behavior. These behaviors also serve unknown purposes and spring from unknown motivations, but like the actions of tribal people from the Trobriand Islands, they raise questions about the sexual aggression of women.

Very few studies have been conducted to determine the prevalence or scope of women's sexual aggression toward men. In much of the classic literature on sexual aggression, it was simply assumed that women were not aggressors or were aggressors very infrequently (Groth & Birnbaum, 1979). In describing what he termed the "male monopoly," Finkelhor (1979) attributed women's lack of sexual aggression to a number of factors. He believed that men engage in more sexually deviant behavior because of incomplete and faulty biological development, because some men become hostile toward women as they reject their symbiotic relationships with their mothers in order to develop appropriate masculinity, and because men make and enforce social rules, in part through sexual dominance, control, and violence toward women. Finkelhor also argued that because women are inferior in strength and because men must play the active role in intercourse, women are basically incapable of raping men. Other authors have argued that some researchers have systematically and purposefully ignored or distorted the data available on sexual violence in order to support their hypothesis that only men are perpetrators and only women are victims of sexual violence (Mould, 1984).

The idea that women can be sexually aggressive is perhaps more likely to surface in the public media rather than the scientific literature. For example, in the much-publicized New York City "Yuppie Murder Trial," self-defense in the face of sexual assault was stipulated by the defense attorney for Robert Chambers in the murder of Jennifer Levin (Pearl, 1986). The defense attempted to show that it was Chambers who was vulnerable in this situation. The basic argument was that Levin was on top of Chambers attempting to force him into having sexual intercourse with her. In the process, she allegedly grabbed Chambers's genitals too hard, causing him to throw her off him in a reflex response to the pain, resulting in her death. The effect of this argument will never be known because the case was settled through a plea bargain while the jury was still in deliberation.

## LITERATURE

The limited research on women who are sexually aggressive toward men focuses on four clusters of respondents: women receiving psychological treatment for a variety of reasons (Friedrich, 1993; Higgs, Canavan, & Meyer, 1992), women referred to treatment through the legal system (Fehrenbach & Monastersky, 1988; Mathews, 1987; Wolfe, 1985), women in prison (Cochran & Drucker, 1984; Condy, Templer, Brown, & Veaco, 1987), and college students (Anderson, 1987; Anderson, 1990; Anderson, 1993; Anderson & Aymami, 1993; Lottes, 1991; Story, 1986). There is also one article that presents some case reports of women on staff at a psychiatric hospital sexually abusing male patients (Laury, 1992). Many of the other important studies of women as sexual initiators or aggressors and men as the receivers of their initiation are being presented by the authors of those studies in this book. Therefore, and because my focus is specifically on reports of women's behaviors, I will not review them here.

One of the challenges of social constructionist thought is to consider variables other than gender that will help explain and provide a depth of analysis for human behavior (White & Kowalski, 1994). Because all the studies cited below were conducted with nonrandom samples of unusual or extreme populations, their results do not represent the general population of women. The results of these studies can, however, yield clues about the variables, other than gender, that warrant further study.

Research based on populations of women in treatment includes a review of recent literature and a case study. The literature review (Friedrich, 1993) supported the contention that sexually abused children are more likely to exhibit increased sexual behavior following the abuse. It is, at times, this behavior that leads to treatment and the discovery of the initial abuse. The case study (Higgs, Canavan, & Meyer, 1992) documented the behavior shift in one 14-year-old girl from sexual victim to sexual offender. Citing their own and other literature, the researchers concluded that being victimized repeatedly, being in a close relationship with the perpetrator, and experiencing more severe sexual abuse is more likely to lead to sexual offending.

Women referred to treatment through the courts have usually committed legal offenses or run away from home or both. Like all of the women discussed here, they are likely victims of sexual, physical, and/or emotional abuse or come from dysfunctional family backgrounds. The three studies that reported on this population (cumulative $N = 63$) supported four characteristics of women as sexual perpetrators. The first characteristic was a higher-than-expected rate of their victims being men (35%); the second was that the majority of the women had been sexually abused as children or young adolescents; the third was that almost all of the women aggressors were friends or acquaintances of the victims; and the fourth was that they were significantly older (5 years or more) than the men they initiated sex with. The women cited several motives for their behavior, including providing sex education, a love affair, fear of a male counterpart, and using the sexual contact as an attempt to stay in or escape a relationship with another man.

The report of women who molested male psychiatric patients (Laury, 1992) offered clinical vignettes as illustrations of the women's motives for their sexual behavior. Their motives included material gain, being seduced by the patient, or being a "good Samaritan" by providing therapy that included sexual contact.

The studies of women in prison included data on 100 women. Of the respondents, 20 were specifically charged with rape (four of their victims were men) and 13 who initiated sexual contact with a man under 16 years old were adults at least 5 years older. The researchers considered past victimization to be a critical variable in women's sexual aggression.

Story (1986) was among the first researchers to obtain self-report data from college women about their sexual initiation or aggression. She used a random sample of all of the students at the University of Northern Iowa to study partner abuse. She found evidence of a higher level of sexual abuse of men by women than previously assumed. In her study she asked students about their experience in giving and receiving partner sexual abuse (a "partner" was defined as a person that one is or has been emotionally involved with in a relationship that may or may not include or have included sexual intimacy). The definitions of abuse ranged from emotional or verbal abuse (including threats) to forced sexual intercourse or physical abuse with or without the use of a weapon. Among the women in her study, approximately 10% reported forcing sexual intimacy of some kind on a partner, including 3.9% who forced sexual intercourse. The author concluded that her data are an underestimate of the real prevalence rates of partner abuse among college students because of her random-sample technique with a high return rate (91.4%) and the fact that people are reluctant to report on behaviors that are perceived negatively.

In another study of college women, Lottes (1991) used data from 398 students to examine the relationships between nontraditional gender roles and sexual "coercion" (e.g., pressuring with continual arguments, making false commitments and promises of love, getting [him] drunk or drugged). The results indicated that women who were less traditional (i.e., initiated and paid for dates) were no more likely to be sexually coercive than women who did not initiate or pay for dates.

I interviewed a 22-year-old woman college student who, during the summer before the interview, had discovered her 15-year-old neighbor "peeping" into her window (Anderson, 1993). She set a trap for him, and after catching him she proceeded to "punish" him for his offense by forcing him to perform oral sex on her on several occasions and also to run errands and wash her car for a 2-month period of time. The abuse ended because she left to go back to college after her summer vacation. During Andrea's interviews, she described Mark as more of a "bookworm type" than a jock. She was certain he was a virgin. Her role as controller and seducer made her feel powerful and alive. She was delighted to have someone under her control, and whenever Mark would be reluctant to do her bidding, renewed threats would weaken his resistance. If Mark had been younger, she said she would have simply called his parents. Despite the fact that she enjoyed the experience, she said that she would be unlikely to repeat it and certainly isn't looking to find another similar situation. She believes that this was simply an unusual life event that will not reoccur. It is possible that these kinds of situational variables play a role in women's sexual victimization of men and also contribute to the lack of reporting of the offenses because the male in the situation has committed an offense as well.

In another study, my colleague and I compared college women's and men's reports of women initiating sexual contact (Anderson & Aymami, 1993). The result was that men reported experiencing women's sexual initiation more frequently than women reported initiating. The exact meaning of these differences is unclear. The respondents were not dating partners, so their experiences could be genuinely different. It could also be that men overreported their experiences because they were confused, misinterpreted their partners' actions, or were self-delusional. Okami (1991) asserts that men, particularly young men, rate women's sexual initiation positively and may overreport. It is also possible that because men were expected to assess women's motives, they attributed each incidence to more than one category on the questionnaire, while women, in assessing their own motives, only attributed each incidence to one category, thus causing the discrepancy. We surmised that traditional gender roles and the tactics (psychological rather than physical) used by women to initiate most sexual contact contributed to the differences in reporting. Women socialized into the "nice girls don't" (Moffatt, 1989) traditional gender role would be less likely to admit certain behaviors and motives involved in initiating sexual contact, particularly those that were blatantly contrary to women's traditional gender roles (e.g., use of power, seduction of a minor, or threat or use of physical force). Traditional gender roles also preserve the notion that men are always interested in and ready for sex with any partner. Women who believe this may not see themselves as the initiator, even if they are. These women would be more likely to underreport their initiation of sexual contact with men.

## THEORY AND RESEARCH QUESTIONS

There is no unified theory or set of theories that can currently be used to explain women's sexual aggression. The studies that have reported on this phenomenon are descriptive in nature and lack any theory-building or -testing component. This lack of theoretical base is not surprising in the study of behaviors that have been denied and ignored until very recently. Several theories have been used to explain male sexual aggression. Some of them hold some promise in the exploration of women's sexual aggression, and others do not.

The hypothesis that rape is the ultimate weapon that men use to maintain social control and dominance over women (Brownmiller, 1975) completely ignores the possibility of women perpetrating sexual victimization. According to this model, men are violent, incapable of negotiating relationships, and uncommunicative with their partners, while women are passive, nurturing, communicative, and nonviolent. Extreme theories like this one do not represent the true diversity of the human community and the behaviors that overlap both genders.

A somewhat related theory is offered by Groth and Birnbaum (1979). His studies of convicted male rapists lead him to conclude that men rape because of feelings of anger or a need for power or control but not for sexual gratification. These conclusions were based on the fact that a large portion of the inmates reported general sexual dysfunctions, as well as a lack of erection, penetration, or orgasm during their sexual assaults. Convicted rapists are certainly not representative of the general population of sexually aggressive men and are probably not representative of rapists as a whole. Theories about the nature of power in sexual relationships and the initiation of sexual contact by women will be addressed by others in this volume.

More recent theories of sexual aggression have attempted to account for the behaviors of a greater portion of men in our society who may never commit a rape (in the traditional sense of using physical force) but who may use verbal pressure, psychological force, or coercion to obtain some kind of sexual activity with a woman without her freely given consent.

The social control–social conflict model (one form of social learning theory) is an attempt to explain sexual aggression in a number of situations by a variety of men who would not necessarily be defined as rapists (Koss, Leonard, Beezley, & Oros, 1985). This model postulates a "sick society" that supports negative attitudes toward women and accepts customs that foster sexual aggression on the part of men (the dominant social force) toward women (those who are dominated). There have been a number of studies that support the argument of social control of sexual violence. This theoretical framework has some possible application to women who are sexually aggressive. As women gain social control, some of them might exercise their social dominance as sexual initiation or aggression.

Social learning theories, like the one noted above, and social constructionism are, I believe, the best theoretical paradigms to explain or predict women's sexual initiation and aggression. While there is no single "social learning" theory, many different social learning and social constructionist theories are particularly relevant to the study of sexual initiation and aggression. Social constructionist theories support the contention that previously reported differences between men and women are a result of social interaction rather than biological determinism. Social learning argues that human behavior, rather than being the result of genetic predetermination, is the result of what we learn throughout our lives.

Two separate studies that analyzed anthropological data from the standard cross-cultural sample published by Textor (1967) provide some support for the social construction of sexually violent behaviors. These data provide information on over 150 of the world's societies, including information on child-rearing practices, sexual behaviors, and physical violence. From the evidence that some societies are significantly more sexually violent than others, Prescott (1975) and Sanday (1981) both concluded that violent behaviors, including rape, are not an inherent part of male or human behavior but are the result of social learning.

The previously cited research by Koss, Leonard, Beezley, and Oros (1985) used scales adapted from the work of Burt (1980) to link attitudes and self-reported behaviors of college men. The men who were most supportive of rape myths and accepting of sex-role stereotypes, who held adversarial beliefs about sexuality, who felt that rape prevention was the woman's responsibility, and who saw the intermingling of aggression and sexuality as normal were more likely to have reported engaging in sexually aggressive behaviors. The results arguably support social learning as relevant in predicting sexual aggression by college men. The next step in supporting a social learning theory explanation of women's sexual aggression has to link women's experiences and attitudes with behavior.

By applying a social learning model to women's sexual aggression, it could be predicted that women who hold stereotypical views of male–female relationships, who are less satisfied with their own sex role, who have experienced sexual abuse in their past, and/or who view sexual relationships as predominately adversarial would be more likely to be sexually aggressive.

I would now like to turn to the three specific questions that I studied with two different samples of college women. The first question was to determine if women engaged in the full range of sexually initiatory and aggressive behaviors attributed to men. The second was to explore the connection between past experience of sexual abuse and women's sexually aggressive behaviors. Past experience of sexual abuse is defined as a minor's experience of sexual contact with someone 5 or more years older or the experience of being forced, coerced, or tricked into sexual activity (Browne & Finkelhor, 1986; Groth, Burgess, & Holmstrom, 1977; Koss et al., 1985).

My final question was to discover the relationship between women's belief that relationships between men and women are essentially adversarial and their willingness to be sexually aggressive toward a heterosexual partner. The measure I chose to use was developed by Burt (1980) in her attempt to discover the psychological, social, and attitudinal correlates of rape. To this end, she developed several attitude scales and correlated them with another scale designed to measure rape myth acceptance. This strategy was based on the assumption that men who accept rape myths that trivialize both rape and the victim will be more likely to engage in tactics to gain sexual access to a woman that could be defined as rape. Among the attitudinal scales found to be highly correlated with rape myth acceptance was Adversarial Sexual Beliefs (ASB). ASB is defined as the belief that "sexual relationships are fundamentally exploitative in that each party is manipulative, sly, cheating, opaque to the other's understanding and not to be trusted" (Burt, 1980, p. 218). Other researchers have subsequently correlated Burt's ASB scale with sexually aggressive behavior on the part of male subjects (Koss et al., 1985) and with the experience of sexual victimization by women (Skelton, 1984).

## STRATEGIES AND PROCEDURES

My research surveys were conducted with women college student volunteers in New Orleans, New Jersey, and New York. The students were all enrolled in undergraduate courses in human sexuality. Each respondent completed Burt's Adversarial Sexual Beliefs scale to measure their attitudes about relationships. Their sexual initiation and aggression was measured by the combined responses to the 24 items that were identical in each of the testing situations taken from an original 26-item Sexually Aggressive Behavior (SAB) scale that I developed. The SAB scale was developed to fully assess a wide range of tactics and motives relative to women's initiating sexual contact. Items ranged from mutually consenting sexual contact (e.g., "How many times have you initiated sexual contact with a man because you both wanted to?") and other motives (e.g., to end another relationship, to gain something from a person in power) through several forms of sexual coercion or abuse (e.g., by using your position of power or authority [boss, teacher, baby-sitter, counselor, or supervisor] or by initiating sexual contact with a minor at least 5 years younger than yourself) and included the use of physical force.

## RESULTS

Of the 476 questionnaires distributed, only 15 were returned with sufficient missing data to render them unusable for statistical analysis. This represents 461 total responses and an overall response rate of 96.8% for the women who were given questionnaires. [The respondents were predominantly single, heterosexual, raised in households headed by professionals or executives, and 21 years old or younger. The respondents scored low on the ASB scale, indicating that they were, as a group, not very adversarial in their beliefs. Approximately 43% of the sample had experienced past sexual abuse of some kind. Additionally, 57% knew of friends or family members who had been abused.

Table 4.1 presents the percentage of respondents answering "yes" to each of the items related to their sexual initiation and aggression. Overall, almost all of the respondents had initiated sexual contact with a man (95.4%). The first four SAB items were intended to establish the existence of noncoercive sexual behaviors and present the questions that I believed to be least threatening first in order to help the respondents gain comfort in answering questions about their sexual behaviors. The frequency of reporting sexually initiatory behavior generally decreased from the first to the last item, which is consistent with the design of the scale. It is interesting to note that even the most extreme behavior was engaged in to some extent by this sample of respondents. Most of the respondents had engaged in mutually consenting sexual contact with a man, had initiated that contact, had overestimated the amount of sexual contact a man wanted to have with them, had attempted to sexually arouse a man to entice him into sexual activity, and had been so sexually aroused themselves that they tried to continue sexual activity even if their male partner was not interested. Conversely, very few women in the sample made threats, used their position of power or authority, used physical force, or threatened a man with a weapon to get him to have sexual contact with them. Approximately half of the sample initiated sexual contact with a man while his judgment was impaired by drugs or alcohol.

Because one purpose of this study was to document the range of college women's sexual aggression, it is important to note that between 26% and 43% of all the women respondents reported

TABLE 4.1. Percentage of Women Responding "Yes" to
Sexually Aggressive Behavior Scale (N = 461)

| Question | % |
|---|---|
| 1. Mutually consenting contact | 98.5 |
| 2. You initiated contact | 95.4 |
| 3. You overestimated partner's desire | 71.7 |
| 4. You attempted to arouse partner | 85.7 |
| 5. You threatened to end relationship | 31.6 |
| 6. You said things you did not mean | 43.0 |
| 7. You pressured with verbal arguments | 34.5 |
| 8. You questioned partner's sexuality | 32.9 |
| 9. To make someone else jealous | 47.0 |
| 10. To hurt someone else | 46.1 |
| 11. To end another relationship | 42.6 |
| 12. To gain something from person in power | 24.8 |
| 13. To express your anger at your partner | 35.0 |
| 14. To retaliate against your partner | 32.3 |
| 15. To gain power or control of partner | 45.7 |
| 16. While he was drunk or stoned | 62.4 |
| 17. By getting him drunk or stoned | 36.5 |
| 18. While he was a minor and you were not | 29.3 |
| 19. By using your position of power/authority | 26.5 |
| 20. By taking advantage of compromising position | 30.6 |
| 21. By threatening to use physical force | 27.8 |
| 22. By using physical force | 20.0 |
| 23. By threatening self-harm | 7.4 |
| 24. By threatening him with a weapon | 8.9 |

engaging in strategies that would be traditionally defined as coercive if applied to male respondents. These strategies include lying,
threatening to end a relationship, and verbal pressure to have sex.
From 26% to 36% of the women reported strategies traditionally
defined as abusive. These strategies are: using your position of power
or authority, getting him drunk or drugged, and taking advantage
of a man while he was in a compromising position. Approximately
20% of the women reported using physical force, 27% the threat
of physical force, and 9% a weapon to obtain sexual contact with a
male partner.

These studies tested two predictions regarding the positive
relationships between a woman's past experience of sexual abuse, her
adversarial sexual beliefs, and her sexually aggressive behavior with
adolescent and adult men. Pearson product–moment correlation

coefficients (*r*) with two-tailed tests of significance were calculated between the scores on the past abuse scale, the ASB scale, and the SAB scale. Results confirmed the predicted relationships. A multiple-regression analysis revealed that the relationship between past abuse and adversarial beliefs was independently related to sexual behavior. In other words, women who held adversarial beliefs about relationships or had experienced sexual abuse in the past were more likely to be sexually aggressive. Subjects with adversarial beliefs and past experience of abuse were no more likely to be sexually aggressive than respondents who met only one of these conditions.

## DISCUSSION AND CONCLUSIONS

According to my research, college women who have been sexually abused in the past and/or those who hold adversarial beliefs about relationships are more likely than their nonabused, nonadversarial counterparts to engage in sexually aggressive behaviors. The data reported here support a social learning model to explain sexual aggression in these samples by substantiating the relationship between personal attitudes, past experience, and current behavior. These findings are important because they provide the first evidence of a relationship between a woman's past experience of sexual abuse, her adversarial beliefs about sexual relationships, and her sexually aggressive behavior.

Sexual arousal as well as other motivations (e.g., a desire to hurt someone else or to gain power or control over a sexual partner) also contribute to women's sexual aggression. The tactics that women use to initiate sexual contact vary considerably. The vast majority of women who initiated sexual contact attempted to sexually arouse their partners; some women used physical force or a weapon to gain sexual access to a man; other women used psychological or verbal pressure in their sexual aggression; and still others took advantage of a man by purposefully altering his judgment with the use of alcohol or drugs. These findings support social constructionist notions of gender differences and underscore the reality of sexual aggression among college students by confirming the fact that women also engage in sexually manipulative behavior that ranges from lying to the use of a weapon. The results also provide important new information about women as aggressors and how they may be similar to, or different from, male aggressors.

The debate over the definitions of sexual behavior will continue in professional, legal, and social settings for a long time to come. Many states and local governments are rewording their definitions of sexually aggressive behaviors in gender-neutral terms, while others continue to maintain legal codes that only allow men to be prosecuted for sexual crimes. In our own profession there is much controversy over and considerable discrepancy between researchers definitions of sexual "coercion," "abuse," or "force." The legitimacy of using definitions traditionally applied to men's behavior for that of women is clearly questionable and ignores power differences between men and women (Irving, 1990).

I would argue that it is indeed an issue of power—power that is socially constructed and learned—that is one of the primary determining factors in sexual aggression. The rarity of sexual aggression among contemporary women is consistent with this argument, as is much of our historical record. Women in many cultures have had little or no power. The concept of women as sexual aggressors is a laughable idea in cultures where women have little power (Anderson, 1986) and may be a uniquely Western phenomenon. As women struggle to become more powerful in our culture, several responses related to sexual aggression are possible. For one, women may be more likely to use their emerging power to fulfill a variety of needs, including the need for sexual contact. Another possibility is that women's lack of ability to gain power efficiently or quickly could lead to frustration that triggers a modeling of the behaviors of their oppressors in order to simulate power or to feel empowered. Farrell (1993) cites a lack of power held by men who commit sexual assaults as their primary motivation. A third possibility is that women will become increasingly tired of being victimized and will move from the defense to the offense. This idea is also consistent with the connection between women's experience of past sexual abuse, their adversarial beliefs about sexual relationships, and their sexual aggression. Whatever conclusions we draw now, it is certain that women's future sexual behavior will be determined by myriad influences that transcend simple gender roles and will require sophisticated research and theoretical approaches to be understood.

# REFERENCES

Anderson, P. (1986). [Unpublished notes.]

Anderson, P. (1987, April). *Women raping men.* Paper presented at the annual meeting of the American Association of Sex Educators, Counselors, and Therapists, New York, NY.

Anderson, P. (1990, November). *Aggressive sexual behavior by females: Incidence, correlates, and implications.* Paper presented at the annual meeting of the Mid-South Educational Research Association, New Orleans, LA.

Anderson, P. (1993). Sexual victimization: It happens to boys too. *Louisiana Association for Health, Physical Education, Recreation, and Dance Journal, 57*(1), 5, 12.

Anderson, P., & Aymami, R. (1993). Reports of female initiation of sexual contact: Male and female differences. *Archives of Sexual Behavior, 22*(4), 335–343.

Browne, A., & Finkelhor, D. (1986). Impact of child sexual abuse: A review of the research. *Psychological Bulletin, 99*(1), 66–77.

Brownmiller, S. (1975). *Against our will: Men, women, and rape.* New York: Simon & Schuster.

Burt, M. (1980). Cultural myths and supports for rape. *Journal of Personality and Social Psychology, 38*(2), 217–230.

Cochran, D., & Drucker, L. (1984). *Women who rape.* Report of the Office of the Commissioner of Probation, Boston, MA.

Condy, S., Templer, D., Brown, R., & Veaco, L. (1987). Parameters of sexual contact of boys with women. *Archives of Sexual Behavior, 16*(5), 379–394.

Farrell, W. (1993). *The myth of male power: Why men are the disposable sex.* New York: Simon & Schuster.

Fehrenbach, P., & Monastersky, C. (1988, January). Characteristics of female adolescent sexual offenders. *American Journal of Orthopsychiatry, 58*(1), 148–151.

Finkelhor, D. (1979). *Sexually victimized children.* New York: Free Press.

Friedrich, W. (1993). Sexual victimization and sexual behavior in children: A review of recent literature. *Child Abuse and Neglect, 17,* 59–66.

Groth, N., & Birnbaum, J. (1979). *Men who rape: The psychology of the offender.* New York: Plenum Press.

Groth, N., Burgess, A., & Holmstrom, L. (1977). Rape, power, anger, and sexuality. *American Journal of Psychiatry, 134*(11), 1239–1243.

Higgs, D., Canavan, M., & Meyer, W. (1992). Moving from the defense to offense: The development of an adolescent female sex offender. *Journal of Sex Research, 29*(1), 131–139.

Irving, J. (1990). From difference to sameness: Gender ideology in sexual science. *Journal of Sex Research, 27*(1), 7–24.

Koss, M., Leonard, K., Beezley, D., & Oros, C. (1985). Nonstranger sexual aggression: A discriminant analysis of the psychological characteristics of undetected offenders. *Sex Roles, 12*(9/10), 981–992.

Laury, G. (1992). When women sexually abuse male psychiatric patients. *Journal of Sex Education and Therapy, 18*(1), 11–16.

Lottes, I. (1991). The relationship between nontraditional gender roles and sexual coercion. *Journal of Psychology and Human Sexuality, 4*(4), 89–109.

Malinowski, B. (1927). *Sex and repression in savage society.* London: Routledge & Kegan Paul.

Mathews, R. (1987). *Female sexual offenders.* Unpublished report, Phase Program, Maplewood, MN.

Moffatt, M. (1989). *Coming of age in New Jersey: College and American culture.* Rutgers, NJ: Rutgers University Press.

Mould, D. (1984). *Men, women, and abused statistics: An examination of frequently referenced wife-battering data.* Unpublished manuscript.

Okami, P. (1991). Self-reports of "positive" childhood and adolescent sexual contacts with older persons: An exploratory study. *Archives of Sexual Behavior, 20*(5), 437–458.

Pearl, M. (1986, November, 13). Chambers: I was raped. *New York Post,* p. 7.

Prescott, J. (1975, November). Body pleasure and the origins of violence. *Bulletin of the Atomic Scientists, 3,* 10–20.

Sanday, P. (1981). The socio-cultural context of rape: A cross-cultural study. *Journal of Social Issues, 37*(4), 5–27.

Skelton, C. (1984). *Correlates of sexual victimization among college women.* Unpublished doctoral dissertation, Auburn, AL: Auburn University.

Story, M. (1986). *Factors affecting the incidence of partner abuse among university students.* Unpublished manuscript, University of Northern Iowa.

Textor, R. (1967). *A cross-cultural summary.* New Haven, CT: HRAF Press.

White, J, & Kowalski, R. (1994). Deconstructing the myth of the nonaggressive woman: A feminist analysis. *Psychology of Women Quarterly, 18,* 487–508.

Wolfe, F. (1985, March). *Twelve female sexual offenders.* Paper presented at the conference on "Next Steps in Research on the Assessment and Treatment of Sexually Aggressive Persons (Paraphiliac)," St. Louis, MO.

# 5

# When the Tables Are Turned: Verbal Sexual Coercion among College Women

MARY E. CRAIG SHEA

Sexual coercion has been documented as a problem both in college settings and in the general population, with 30–77% of women reporting having unwanted sexual contact (e.g., Burkhart & Stanton, 1988; Muehlenhard & Linton, 1987). Characteristics of male perpetrators and female victims have been well described, as have the types of situations in which coercion typically occurs, the thought processes associated with the offense, and the feelings of the participants afterward (for a review, see Craig, 1990). In the course of conducting coercion research, however, one question has arisen repeatedly that has not been addressed in the literature, namely: How frequently are the roles in sexual coercion reversed? That is, do women pressure men to have intercourse against their will and, if so, what are the characteristics of these women?

Anecdotally, we hear of cases in which men have been pressured to have sexual relationships they did not want, but it is impossible to know from these limited—and frequently sensationalized—accounts whether they are "typical" cases. Also, the attention has been primarily on the victims of female sexual coercion. Little has been written about the female coercers themselves.

With this increase in public and media interest in sexual harassment and coercion, new realities and myths have come to light. It is important in the early stages of our research that we define which of our beliefs are myths and which are facts.

This chapter describes two studies: The first is an investigation of the prevalence of sexual coercion of men by women and an initial investigation of the characteristics, feelings, and motivations of coercive women; the second is a further investigation of the histories, beliefs, arousal patterns, and social behavior of identified coercive women.

# STUDY 1

Participants were 171 female college students at a large southeastern university. All participants completed a questionnaire on their demographics and dating history and four instruments: the Sexual Experiences Survey (SES; Koss & Oros, 1982), the Sexual Attitudes Scale (SAS; Craig, Follingstad, Franklin, & Kalichman, 1988; see Appendix); the Rape Arousal Inventory (RAI; Briere, Corne, Runtz, & Malamuth, 1984), and the Sexual Experience Checklist (SEC; Craig et al., 1988). Because these scales were originally designed for men, the wording was changed on each to reverse gender references.

The SES is a 12-item self-report questionnaire that assesses participants' experience with consensual, coerced, and forced intercourse. Women were classified, based on their responses to this survey, as being sexually inexperienced, consensually experienced only, verbally coercive, or sexually assaultive. Verbal coercion was defined minimally as having sexual intercourse with a man "when [she] knew *he* did not want to" by saying things she did not mean, making false promises, or just going ahead, even though he said not to.

The SAS is a 19-item factor-analytically derived scale designed to differentiate between sexually coercive and noncoercive individuals. It has previously been used with coercive and noncoercive men to assess exploitative tendencies in relationships, acceptance of force as a means to obtain intercourse, and beliefs that heterosexual relationships are adversarial by nature (Craig, Kalichman, &

Follingstad, 1989). This scale was reanalyzed for the current study, resulting in three factors for women: Adversity/Force, Exploitation, and Nontraditional Sexual Beliefs.

The RAI was administered to assess which aspects of a hypothetical rape the participant (as perpetrator) would find arousing. It asks, "If it were possible for you to force a man to have sex with you where no one would ever know and you wouldn't be caught, what parts (if any) would you find arousing or exciting?" This 14-item scale contains three subscales: Sex/Subjugation, Hatred/Degradation, and Power/Domination. This instrument has been used to effectively discriminate between sexually aggressive and nonaggressive men (Briere et al., 1984).

The final instrument, the SEC, is a list of 23 adjectives describing feelings a person may experience during a sexual encounter (e.g., aroused, full of love, drunk). Participants responded in a yes/no format as to whether they were experiencing each of the feelings at the time of a particular sexual encounter. In order to control for the choice of partner described by the women, they were asked to answer all questions in reference to the sexual partner they had known least well, described as a stranger/acquaintance, a first or second date, an occasional date, or a steady date/fiancé.

The mean age of all participants was 18.6 ($SD$ = 1.3). Eighty percent of the women were white; 65% were in their freshman year. The sexually active women had an average of 1.1 sexual partners in the past month and 4.9 sexual encounters in the past month. Participants were grouped into four levels of sexual experience, based on the SES. Of the 171 female undergraduates completing the questionnaires, 18% were classified as being sexually inexperienced, 62% reported having had only consensual sexual experiences, and 19% were classified as having verbally coerced a partner into a sexual encounter. Only two participants were classified as being sexually assaultive; this group was therefore omitted from further analyses.

The groups did not differ on demographic variables, with the exception of their number of years of dating experience. The sexually inexperienced women had an average of 3.5 years of dating experience, while the noncoercive women had 4.7 years and the coercive women had an average of 6.3 years.

When the women were asked to describe the types of relationships in which they had sex, differences were found between the coercive and noncoercive groups. As expected, most of the women in both groups had sexual encounters only in established relationships. However, there was a larger percentage of coercive women (41% vs. 29%) who had also had sex with first or second dates, occasional dates, and strangers. These results are displayed in Table 5.1.

The SAS and RAI both showed significant differences between the coercive and noncoercive groups. Coercive women were more likely to report sexual arousal to the physical sensations on the RAI Sex/Subjugation subscale (i.e., the feeling of his naked body, the act of sexual intercourse), the novelty of the situation (i.e., having sex with a stranger, trying a "kinky" sexual act with a man, the chance to have sex in an unusual situation) and control and power on the RAI Power/Domination subscale (i.e., the knowledge that he was totally helpless, the act of overpowering a man, feeling him struggle) than noncoercive women. There was also a slight difference on the SAS Nontraditional Sexual Beliefs subscale (i.e., it is acceptable for a woman to pay for a date; I do not lose respect for a man who has sexual relationships without any emotional involvement; if a man gets drunk at a party and has sex with a woman he just met there, he should be considered fair game for other women who want to have sex with him whether he wants to or not), with coercive women being less accepting of traditional sex roles. No significant differences were found on the SAS Exploitation or SAS Adversity/Force subscales or the RAI Hatred/Degradation subscale. Mean scores for each group on the SAS and RAI are presented in Table 5.2.

The last instrument examined the feelings experienced by the women at the time of a particular sexual encounter. Frequency tabulations were calculated for each of the 23 feelings listed on the SEC. For the noncoercive group, the five most frequently endorsed

**TABLE 5.1. Earliest Stage of Relationship Development in Which Women Reported Having Engaged in Sexual Intercourse**

|  | Noncoercive (N = 106) | Coercive (N = 32) |
|---|---|---|
| Stranger/acquaintance | 9% | 15% |
| First or second date | 8% | 4% |
| Occasional date | 12% | 22% |
| Steady date/fiancé | 71% | 59% |

TABLE 5.2. Noncoercive and Coercive Women's Mean Scores (and Standard Deviations) on the Sexual Attitudes Scale and Rape Arousal Inventory

|  | Inexperienced ($N$ = 31) | Noncoercive ($N$ = 106) | Coercive ($N$ = 32) |
|---|---|---|---|
| SAS |  |  |  |
| Adversity/Force | 16.7 | 17.4 | 17.2 |
|  | (4.0) | (3.9) | (4.0) |
| Exploitation | 8.1 | 8.0 | 8.3 |
|  | (1.1) | (1.0) | (1.5) |
| Nontraditional Sexual | 11.6 | 12.3 | 12.9[a] |
| Beliefs | (1.8) | (2.4) | (1.8) |
| RAI |  |  |  |
| Sex/Subjugation | 10.8 | 11.7 | 13.6[*] |
|  | (4.6) | (4.5) | (4.4) |
| Hatred/Degradation | 5.1 | 4.8 | 5.0 |
|  | (2.5) | (1.4) | (1.9) |
| Power/Domination | 6.1 | 6.0 | 7.3[*] |
|  | (2.8) | (2.4) | (2.6) |

[a]Nonsignificant trend, $p < .07$
[*]$p < .05$.

items were *sexy* (44%), *needing affection* (42%), *aroused* (41%), *attractive* (41%), and *drunk* (37%). For the coercive group, the five most frequently endorsed items were *very sexually attracted to him* (52%), *powerful* (44%), *horny* (44%), *sexy* (44%), and *needing affection* (44%).

# STUDY 2

Participants were 261 college women who completed the following measures: a questionnaire about their own dating patterns and experiences with physical aggression and sexual coercion in relationships; the Self-Monitoring Scale (SMS; Snyder, 1974); the Social–Sexual Desirability Scale of the Multiphasic Sex Inventory (SSDS; Nichols & Molinder, 1984); and a questionnaire on their beliefs about the acceptability of forced intercourse in various situations.

The SMS is an 18-item measure of personality stability across social situations. Subjects are classified as low self-monitors if they remain much the same across a wide variety of social settings.

Conversely, they are classified as high self-monitors if they adapt their behavior to fit individual situations. Reliability of this scale has been reported by Snyder (1987).

The SSDS consists of 35 items in a true–false format and assesses participants' willingness to admit sexual feelings.

Participants ranged in age from 17 to 68, with a mean age of 19.4 years (*SD* = 4.92). Ninety-six percent were single, and 84% were currently involved in dating relationships.

As defined by the questionnaire, which asked, "How many times have you ever had sexual intercourse with a person when you knew *they* didn't want to, by saying things you didn't mean, making false promises, or just going ahead, even though they said not to," 4% of the women surveyed had a history of verbal sexual coercion and 1% were classified as sexually assaultive.

Coercive women were more likely than noncoercive women to have been recipients of physical force by their parents during childhood. They were also more likely to have used nonsexual physical force (e.g. pushed, slapped, shoved, punched, kicked, thrown an object at, threatened with a weapon) in their own relationships with men.

Coercers were more likely to have said "no" but meant "yes" to sexual intercourse (i.e., "for some reason you indicated that you didn't want to *although you had every intention to and were willing to engage in sexual intercourse*"). In fact, none of the women who had never said "no" and meant "yes" were coercive themselves. Not surprisingly, then, coercive women were more likely to believe that forced intercourse by a woman of a man is acceptable in some situations. These situations are described in Table 5.3.

Similarly, coercive women were more likely to report having been coerced by a man to have sexual intercourse when they did not want to but gave in because of persistent pressure and arguments. This may have been in part due to their belief systems, as 11% of coercive women, but 0% of noncoercive women, believed that the man should have the "final say" in how far sexual contact should progress.

On the SMS, coercive women tended to be higher self-monitors than noncoercive women, meaning that they are more likely to mold their personalities to the expectations of those around them.

Their dating patterns differed also. Whereas most noncoercive women described their first date with their most recent dating

TABLE 5.3. Situations in Which Women Believe That Forced Intercourse by a Woman of a Man Is Acceptable, by Sexual History

|  | Sexually inexperienced ($N = 50$) | Consensual experience only ($N = 197$) | Coercive ($N = 14$) |
|---|---|---|---|
| Both partners have willingly taken off their clothes | 19% | 27% | 50%** |
| He has touched her genitals | 6% | 21% | 34%* |
| He has performed oral sex on her | 6% | 21% | 34%* |
| She has performed oral sex on him | 6% | 17% | 34%* |

*$p < .05$; **$p < .01$.

partner as going out to dinner or to some other structured event, coercive women more frequently described these dates as going to a party and then back to her apartment. Further, coercive women were more likely to have used alcohol on their first dates with their current partners and to have gone out with friends rather than alone.

Finally, as measured by the SSDS, the coercive women were more willing to admit common sexual feelings and desires (i.e., I like to look at sexy pictures; X-rated movies would interest me; when a woman is with an attractive man, her thoughts turn to sex).

## DISCUSSION

Although verbal sexual coercion by women is not as common as that by men, it is a behavior reported by some college women. The prevalence data vary considerably, depending on how the question is asked, but included 4–19% of the women in the current studies.

Although the number of coercers varied, the characteristics of the women in these two studies were similar. They can be described by their personal histories, their belief systems, their behavior, and their arousal patterns. In each of these categories, coercive women differ from traditional or stereotyped depictions of women. The results of these studies are based upon relatively small numbers of coercive women, and they cannot be generalized to all college women. However, if I were to draw a picture of coercive college women, they are more aggressive and power-oriented; they tend to view relationships, and sex in particular, as a game or means of gaining advantage; and feelings of tenderness and love are not necessary components of their sexual encounters.

Coercive women do not differ from noncoercive women in age but have had more experience with dating. They do not appear to be more promiscuous or sexually active, but they do begin having sex with their partners earlier in their relationships. Violence and game playing have long been a part of their most intimate relationships, beginning with their parents and continuing into their romantic liaisons.

These women can also be distinguished from their noncoercive peers by their attitudes about equality. They are more likely to believe that women's traditional roles are constricting and to dismiss them as not being applicable to themselves. This holds true as well for their ideas about sexual equality. They believe that it is both acceptable and appropriate for a woman to have sexual thoughts and desires and for her to act on those desires in a direct way. If directness does not work, however, they may resort to emotional manipulation and other forms of coercion.

These coercive women do not seem to believe that their coercive behavior is necessarily bad or wrong. They are more likely to acknowledge having had sex when they did not want to, and they feel that even forcing someone to have sexual relations against their will is acceptable at times. Thus, it seems that they simply expect and accept coercion and force as a natural part of some relationships. These findings are especially interesting in the light of slowly changing sex roles for men, who have learned to become more sensitive, emotional, and gentle in the past several years. Meanwhile, a certain subgroup of women are becoming more detached, pragmatic, and forceful in their relationships.

Coercive and noncoercive women differ in their social as well as sexual relationships. Coercive women are highly attuned to the expectations of others and are able to change their own approach to fit various situations. They describe themselves as being socially flexible and able to put others at ease. They tend to be more dramatic in their style than noncoercers and like to be the center of attention. In line with this, they frequently describe their first dates with a new partner as going to a party or other social gathering with friends where alcohol is consumed. Disinhibited and happy after the party, coercive women are more likely than their noncoercive peers to invite their dates back to their apartments.

Perhaps most interesting, though, is that when women coerce their dates, they feel differently than noncoercers do in sexual situations. The consensual group describes their feelings in romantic and relationship-oriented terms (e.g. "sexy," "attractive"). Their sexual behavior is a reflection of how they feel about being part of a couple and how that makes them feel about themselves. Even their negative descriptors seem to reflect this: When the relationship has not been what they "needed" it to be to justify the level of sexual activity, they report having been drunk, thus removing the responsibility from themselves. The coercive women, on the other hand, seem to be more goal-directed in their quests—they describe being very sexually attracted to the man, being "horny," and feeling powerful. Their sexual behavior is an indication of lust and suggests less concern about the relationship itself. Sex is the goal, not romance. When fantasizing about forcing a man to have sex, they are also aroused by the elements of raw sex and power. This finding provides support for the feminist view of sexual aggression as being driven by power and control rather than sex. Verbal coercion, for these women, has aspects of both rape and seduction, and therefore seems to lie near the center of a continuum between consensual sexual expression and rape, as has been hypothesized with coercive men.

The current studies looked only at verbally coercive women, as there were too few sexually aggressive women in these samples to draw conclusions about them. Future research should examine the characteristics and thought processes of women who rape, to evaluate the role of power and control in their behavior, as well as their beliefs, interpersonal dynamics, and thought processes.

Further research is also needed to more precisely determine the prevalence of verbal sexual coercion in women and to define other characteristics of these women, the situations they choose and create for themselves, and the consequences of their actions. Sexually aggressive and coercive men have been shown to have complex cognitive distortions. It remains unclear whether coercive women will demonstrate a similar pattern or whether they will have a unique phenomenology. It will also be interesting to examine trends in sexual coercion as our society continues to evolve, noting how social changes affect the sexual behavior and expression of women.

## APPENDIX. Sexual Attitudes Scale

Adversity/Force factor      Reliability (alpha) = .71

1. Many men are so demanding sexually that a woman just can't satisfy them.
2. A woman's got to show a man who's boss right from the start or she'll end up sorry.
3. Men are usually sweet until they've caught a woman, but then they let their true self show.
4. A lot of men seem to get pleasure in putting a woman down.
5. Being roughed up by a woman is sexually stimulating to many men.
6. Many times a man will pretend he doesn't want to have sexual intercourse because he doesn't want to seem promiscuous, but he's really hoping the woman will force him.
7. Sometimes the only way a woman can get a man turned on is to use force.
8. Many men have an unconscious wish to be raped and may then unconsciously set up a situation in which they are likely to be attacked.

Exploitation factor      Reliability (alpha) = .59

9. If I could be assured that no one would know and that I could in no way be punished, I would be likely to rape a man.
10. I would attempt to intoxicate a man with alcohol or other drugs to get him to have sex with me.
11. I have had sexual intercourse with a man who a friend recommended as "easy."
12. Two people should have sex only if they are in a long-term committed relationship.
13. There is nothing wrong with casual sex.

Nontraditional Sexual Beliefs factor      Reliability (alpha) = .49

14. A man who is stuck up and thinks he is too good to talk to women on the street deserves to be taught a lesson.
15. When I see an attractive man, I enjoy imagining what he would be like in bed.

*Note.* All responses are based on a 4-point Likert scale, ranging from "disagree" to "agree," with no midpoint selection.

16. My parent encouraged me to become sexually active.
17. It is acceptable for the woman to pay for the date.
18. I have no respect for a man who engages in sexual relationships without any emotional involvement.
19. If a man gets drunk at a party and has intercourse with a woman he's just met there, he should be considered "fair game" to other females at the party who want to have sex with him, whether he wants to or not.

## REFERENCES

Briere, J., Corne, S., Runtz, M., & Malamuth, N. (1984, August). *The rape arousal inventory: Predicting actual and potential sexual aggression in a university population.* Paper presented at the annual meeting of the American Psychological Association, Toronto, Ontario, Canada.

Burkhart, B., & Stanton, A. (1988). Sexual aggression in acquaintance relationships. In G. Russell (Ed.), *Violence in intimate relationships.* Great Neck, NY: PMA.

Craig, M. (1990). Coercive sexuality in dating relationships: A situational model. *Clinical Psychology Review, 10,* 395–423.

Craig, M., Follingstad, D., Franklin, B., & Kalichman, S. (1988). *Coercive sexual behavior among college students: Who, why, and how often?* Paper presented at the meeting of the Southeastern Psychological Association, New Orleans, LA.

Craig, M., Kalichman, S., & Follingstad, D. (1989). Verbal coercive sexual behavior among college students. *Archives of Sexual Behavior, 18,* 421–434.

Koss, M., & Oros, C. (1982). Sexual Experiences Survey: A research instrument investigating sexual aggression and victimization. *Journal of Consulting and Clinical Psychology, 50,* 455–457.

Muehlenhard, C., & Linton, M. (1987). Date rape and sexual aggression in dating situations: Incidence and risk factors. *Journal of Counseling Psychology, 34,* 186–196.

Nichols, H., & Molinder, I. (1984). *Multiphasic sex inventory manual.* (Available from the authors, 437 Bowes Drive, Tacoma, WA 98466)

Snyder, M. (1974). The self-monitoring of expressive behavior. *Journal of Personality and Social Psychology, 30,* 526–537.

Snyder, M. (1987). *Public appearances, private realities: The psychology of self-monitoring.* New York: Freeman.

# 6

## Why Some Sexual Assaults Are Not Committed by Men: A Biosocial Analysis

### LEE ELLIS

At least since the publication of Susan Brownmiller's (1975) *Against Our Will,* the feminist theory has been the most popular social science explanation for rape (Smith & Bennett, 1985). Above all else, this theory has challenged the assumption that most rapes are sexually motivated (reviewed by Ellis, 1989, p. 10). Some feminist writers have gone so far as to declare rape a "pseudosexual act" (Groth, 1979; Groth & Burgess, 1978). Rather than being sexually motivated, from the feminist perspective, rapes are offenses in which aggressive sexuality is used by men to intimidate and humiliate women, thereby keeping women in subordinate and subservient relationships. To quote Brownmiller, "[Rape] is nothing more or less than a conscious process of intimidation by which *all men* keep *all women* in a state of fear" (1975, p. 5, emphasis in original).

Elsewhere, I have pointed to problems with the feminist theory (Ellis, 1989, p. 19; 1991, p. 632; see also McConaghy, 1993). One problem is that it implies, as Brownmiller states, that rapists will be consciously aware of the nonsexual nature of their acts. The evidence, however, points in the opposite direction. Responses to anonymous questionnaires indicate that most rapists recall that their primary motivation actually *was* sexual (reviewed by Ellis, 1989, p. 22). Although rapists could be lying on this matter, another possibility is that the feminist theory is in error.

Another problem with the feminist theory is its implication that rapes and other sexual assaults that may not meet all legal standards of rape, would be offenses that few if any women would perpetrate. This chapter will show that while the majority of rapes and other sexual assaults are committed by men, a substantial minority are not.

A few years ago, I proposed an alternative to the feminist theory (Ellis, 1989, 1991). This alternative theory explicitly asserts that there are complex links between power, control, and sexual relationships between men and women. It also contends that some sexual assaults, especially those involving a minimum of physical force, will be committed by women against men. Before reviewing evidence pertaining to this latter hypothesis, I will briefly describe this theory.

## THE BIOSOCIAL (SYNTHESIZED) THEORY
## OF SEXUAL ASSAULT

Because the theory I have proposed combines biological with social learning concepts, I have termed it a biosocial (or synthesized) theory (Ellis, 1989, p. 55; 1991, 1993). It can be best summarized in terms of the following four propositions.

*Proposition 1: The motivation to engage in sexual aggression is the result of two drives, the sex drive and the drive to possess and control.* Because of similar evolved neurological processes, it is asserted that humans share with many other animals a sex drive and a tendency to behave possessively toward reproductively significant environmental resources, including members of the opposite sex. In humans, several studies have shown that men and women are frequently very possessive toward one another in terms of exclusive control over sexual behavior (Dutton & Painter, 1981, p. 145; Eibl-Eibesfeldt, 1987, p. 24; Stets & Pirog-Good, 1987, p. 245).

*Proposition 2: Natural selection has favored males with a stronger sex drive, while it has favored females with greater sexual restraint until after a prospective sex partner has demonstrated commitment to a long-term cooperative relationship.* The reason males on average have evolved a stronger sex drive than females is that the main delimiter on a male's reproductive potential is the number of females with whom he can mate. This is not true for females. For them, a major delimiter is having to bear and rear offspring without help. Thus, females will be favored for restricting their sexual interactions to males who appear willing to help care for offspring. The disparity in these two optimal approaches to reproduction bring the average male and female into conflict (Low, 1990).

*Proposition 3: Although the motivation for sexual assault is essentially unlearned, the actual tactics are learned primarily by continual experimentation during courtship and minimally through culturally acquired attitudes.* During dating and other circumstances when sexual experimentation is possible, members of both sexes try a variety of tactics for helping to satiate their sexual desires. Some of these tactics will almost certainly involve the use of deception and pressure. If these tactics are rewarded in terms of progress toward sexual intimacy, the probability of their being used in even more extreme forms in the future is increased.

*Proposition 4: Due to variations in brain exposure to sex hormones, especially testosterone, individuals will vary in the strength of their sex drives and in their sensitivity to pain and to victim suffering. Individuals with the strongest sex drives and the lowest sensitivity will be most prone toward learning sexual aggression.* Brains that are exposed to high levels of testosterone following puberty, in combination with high levels of testosterone's main metabolite, estradiol, before birth, are hypothesized to have a strong sex drive and low sensitivity to most environmental stimuli. The regions of the brain that appear to be most affected in this regard are in and around the hypothalamus and limbic system (Ellis, 1991, p. 634). According to the biosocial theory, lowered sensitivity to environmental stimuli will increase the probability of individuals being insensitive to the pain and distress experienced by victims of sexual aggression. It is also worth noting that testosterone acts outside the nervous system as well as within. Outside the nervous system, testosterone can affect both musculature and growth rates (Mills, Shiono, Shapiro, Crawford, & Rhoads, 1986; Kemper, 1990, p. 30; Halpern, Udry, Campbell, Suchindran, & Mason, 1994; Bergada & Bergada, 1995), which could also affect the ability of males to successfully use force in social interactions.

# A MODEL OF THE BIOSOCIAL THEORY

A model of the biosocial theory of sexual assault is presented in Figure 6.1. Along the bottom of the $x$-axis are the main postulated neurohormonal causes of sexual assault. At the top of the figure are represented the learning variables that the theory maintains are directly causing individuals to use both deceptive and forceful tactics to satiate their sex drive and their drive to possess and control sex partners.

The theory hypothesizes that as one moves along the $x$-axis from left to right, the probability of learning deceptive copulatory tactics begins to be "significant" about a third of the way along the axis. About two-thirds of the way along the $x$-axis the probability of learning actual force as a copulatory tactic begins to be "significant." By the time one reaches the extreme right end, the probability is almost certain that both deceptive and forced copulatory tactics will be readily learned.

Turning attention to the two distribution curves shown in Figure 6.1, the biosocial theory assumes that both men and women are normally distributed with respect to the characteristics identified as varying along the $x$-axis. However, the sexes are hypothesized to differ in two respects. One is that men are assumed to be more widely dispersed than women regarding the traits identified along the $x$-axis. This assumption coincides with evidence that males are more dispersed than are females for a wide variety of behavioral and physiological variables (see Ellis, 1989, p. 84; Sattler, 1988; Koskinen & Martelin, 1994). Second, the averages for the two sexes are hypothesized to be different, with males having a stronger sex drive, a greater desire to possess and control multiple sex partners, and less sensitivity to pain and the suffering of others. In other words, because of the greater exposure of their brains to testosterone (and ultimately because of natural selection), men are further to the right along the $x$-axis than women.

The biosocial theory of sexual assault needs to be carefully tested in ways delineated elsewhere (Ellis, 1989, p. 81). In the present context, only one prediction will be scrutinized: That sexual assault will not be strictly an offense that men commit against women. Instead, the biosocial theory hypothesizes that a substantial minority of offenders should be women. As shown in Figure 6.1, the proportion of female offenders and male victims should become less

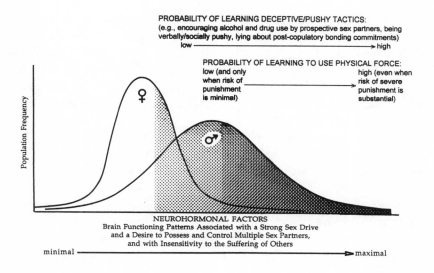

PROBABILITY OF LEARNING DECEPTIVE/PUSHY TACTICS:
(e.g., encouraging alcohol and drug use by prospective sex partners, being verbally/socially pushy, lying about post-copulatory bonding commitments)
low ──────────────────────────────────→ high

PROBABILITY OF LEARNING TO USE PHYSICAL FORCE:
low (and only                              high (even when
when risk of _____                risk of severe
punishment                                 punishment is
is minimal)                                substantial)

Population Frequency

♀

♂

NEUROHORMONAL FACTORS
Brain Functioning Patterns Associated with a Strong Sex Drive
and a Desire to Possess and Control Multiple Sex Partners,
and with Insensitivity to the Suffering of Others

minimal ──────────────────────────────────▶ maximal

FIGURE 6.1. A diagrammatic model of the biosocial theory of sexual assault.

and less as one moves from the least physically violent to the most physically violent cases. I will now review evidence bearing on this hypothesis.

## EVIDENCE OF THE RELATIVE INCIDENCE OF FEMALE-TO-MALE SEXUAL ASSAULTS

Following common practice, the term "sexual assault" will be used here to refer to all physical as well as verbal and social threats or use of pressure or force to initiate intimate sexual contact (Sorenson, Stein, Siegel, Golding, & Burnam, 1987, p. 1156). The degree of pressure or force can vary all the way from constantly nagging dates to the use of weapons and inflicting physical injuries. The strictly nonphysical examples of sexual assault would probably be best described as "nonconsensual sexual activity" (Moore, Nord, & Peterson, 1989), thereby reserving the word "rape" for examples of sexual assault involving the use (or threat) of actual physical force (Ellis, 1989, p. 1).

Although most studies of sexual assault have essentially assumed that only women are victims and only men are perpetrators (see, e.g., Kirkpatrick & Kanin, 1957; Johnson, 1980; Kanin, 1983, 1984; Koss & Oros, 1982; Russell, 1984; Koss, Gidycz, & Wisniewski, 1987), 19 studies published since 1980 were located that made it possible to estimate the proportion of each sex victimized by sexual assault. The results of these studies are summarized in Table 6.1.

As one can see from the second column of Table 6.1, all but one of the studies were conducted in the United States, the exception being a study of teenagers in England (Hartless, Ditton, Nair, & Phillips, 1995). Seven of the studies were based on samples of university students, with the remaining studies coming from a variety of other samples and a few from entire populations. Wherever possible, instances of men being sexually assaulted by other men were excluded from the proportions that are represented in Table 6.1.

The third column of Table 6.1 describes the nature of the assaults, using abbreviated phrases that are close to the descriptions of the offenses given in the original reports. Some of the descriptions were very broad, such as "was sexually assaulted," while others were quite specific, such as "physically harmed/threatened in order to have sex."

The observed proportions of male victims (or female perpetrators) are presented in the fourth column. The percentages represent the proportion of all victims who were male and/or the proportion of all perpetrators who were female for a particular category of sexual assault. Some of the studies provided information about two or more types of sexual assaults, making it possible to derive a total of 32 different proportions from the 19 studies.

To make it easier to digest the 32 proportions of male victims (or female perpetrators) identified in the fourth column of Table 6.1, I have also prepared Figure 6.2. It arrays the proportions in descending order from left to right along the *x*-axis.

As the reader can see either by examining the fourth column of Table 6.1 or Figure 6.2, the proportions of male victims (or female perpetrators) varied tremendously, all the way from a high of 57% to a low of 0%. If the biosocial theory of sexual assault is correct, the assaults with high proportions of male victims (or female perpetrators) will be those primarily involving the use of verbal/social pressure and those with high proportions of female victims (or

## TABLE 6.1. Proportion of Sexual Assaults in Which Men Were Victimized by Women

| Study | Sample (or population) | Description of offenses sampled | Proportion of male victims |
|---|---|---|---|
| Anonymous (1989) | Los Angeles residents | Self-report of having been forced to have sex | 33% male victims |
| Calderwood (1987, p. 53) | Callers to a rape crisis hot line at New York University | Victims of forced sex | 20% male victims |
| Chadwick & Top (1993, p. 62) | Utah Mormon teenagers | Pressured to have sex in a dating situation | 50% male victims |
| Ellis, Hoffman, & Burke (1990, p. 1210) | Students at Minot State University, North Dakota | Fought to the point of injury in order to have sex with a member of the opposite sex | 9% female perpetrators |
| Frazier (1993) | Patients in a Minneapolis hospital emergency room | Sexual assault victims | 5.1% male victims |
| Groth & Burgess (1980, p. 806) | Calls to Boston Police Department | Reports of sexual assault victimization to the police | 1% male victims |
| | Calls to Philadelphia Rape Crisis Center | Reports of sexual assault victimization to counselors | 6% male victims |
| Hall & Flannery (1984) | Teenagers in Milwaukee, Wisconsin | Experienced forced sex or were threatened for the purpose of having sex | 14.3% male victims |
| Hartless et al. (1995, p. 119) | Teenagers in England | Victims of sexual harassment or threats | 25.8% male victims |
| Kaufman, Divasto, Jackson, Voorhees, & Christy (1980) | Calls to a New Mexico rape crisis clinic | Victims of sexual assault | 5.7% male victims |
| Laumann, Gagnon, Michael, & Michaels (1994, p. 335) | Representative sample of the United States | Victims of sexual assault by a member of the opposite sex | 1.5% male victims |

(continued)

111

**TABLE 6.1.** (*continued*)

| Study | Sample (or population) | Description of offenses sampled | Proportion of male victims |
|---|---|---|---|
| Lott, Reilly, & Howard (1982, pp. 302, 303, 312) | Students and personnel at the University of Rhode Island | Experienced sexual assault on campus<br>  Without penetration<br>  With penetration<br>Experienced sexual assault off campus<br>  Without penetration<br>  With penetration<br>Sexual assault known to have occurred to someone other than subject<br>  Without penetration<br>  With penetration<br>Committed sexual assault | <br>6.8% female perpetrators<br>0% female perpetrators<br><br>3.3% female perpetrators<br>0% female perpetrators<br><br><br>3.7% female perpetrators<br>0% female perpetrators<br>9.0% female perpetrators |
| Muehlenhard & Cook (1988) | Students at the University of Kansas | Unwanted sexual intercourse | 57% male victims |
| Russell (1984, p. 67) | United States | Arrested for forcible rape | 0.8% female perpetrators |
| Rouse (1988, p. 316) | Students at the University of Texas at Arlington | From verbal pressure to have sex to overt sexual aggression | 48% male victims |
| Sigelman, Berry, & Wiles (1984, p. 538) | Students at Eastern Kentucky University | Victim of sexual aggression<br>Admitting to committing sexual aggression | 37.5% male victims<br>14.3% female perpetrators |
| Sorenson & Siegel (1992, p. 96) | Los Angeles, general population | Physically harmed/threatened to have sex<br>Verbally pressured to have sex | 22.6% male victims<br>56.3% male victims |
| Struckman-Johnson (1988, p. 297) | Students at the University of South Dakota | Physically forced to have sex<br>Some potential for or threat of physical pressure to have sex<br>Verbally pressured to have sex | 4.2% male victims<br>11.8% male victims<br><br>21.8% male victims |
| U.S. Department of Justice (1989, p. 297) | United States general population | Self-reported victimization in nationwide survey (National Crime Victimization Survey) | 7% male victims |

*Note.* The percentages represent the proportion of all victims who were male and/or the proportion of all perpetrators who were female for a particular category of sexual assault.

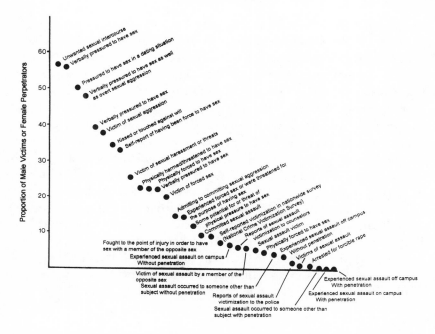

FIGURE 6.2. Proportion of sexual assault victims who are male or perpetrators who are female according to the nature of the sexual assault.

male perpetrators) will be those involving the greatest use of physical force.

Eight of the proportions exceeded 30% male victims (or female perpetrators). Consistent with the biosocial hypothesis, most of these eight proportions either pertained to the use of verbal/social pressure (e.g., "pressured to have sex in a dating situation") or were too generic to specifically interpret as to the nature of the sexual assault (e.g., "victim of sexual aggression," "unwanted sexual intercourse"). When one moves to proportions in the range of 5 to 25% male victims (or female perpetrators), most of the descriptions involve mild use of physical pressure or force (e.g., "physically harmed/threatened to have sex," "experienced forced sex or were threatened for the purpose of having sex") or again are generic in depicting the nature of the assault (e.g., "admitted to sexual aggression," "committed sexual assault").

According to the biosocial theory, it is primarily only in sexual assaults where a great degree of physical force is used that the proportion of male victims (or female perpetrators) should be extremely low. Support for this hypothesis comes from examining the descriptions given for the sexual assaults with the lowest proportions of male victims (or female perpetrators). For sexual assaults involving 5% or fewer male victims (or female perpetrators), one finds sexual assaults that are reported to police or for which individuals are actually arrested and imprisoned, although there are also a few fairly generic descriptions, such as "experienced sexual assault" and "victims of sexual assault." In other words, unlike nonphysical sexual assaults, which women engage in at fairly high rates, few physical sexual assaults (i.e., most prosecutable rapes) are committed by women. Although it may be a coincidence, it seems worth noting that even the slope of the curve that would best fit the 32 observation points represented in Figure 6.2 closely matches the upper halves of two normal curves represented in Figure 6.1. This would coincide with theoretical predictions if one assumes that the points represent increasing degrees of physical force being employed.

## DISCUSSION AND CONCLUSIONS

The purpose of this chapter was to assess evidence pertaining to the relative contribution of women to sexual assault. This investigation was inspired by the continuing controversy over the motivation for sexual assault. If the feminist theory is correct, rapes (as well as sexual assaults not meeting legal standards) should primarily lack sexual motivation. Instead, these acts should be among the methods used by men in patriarchal societies to keep women in subservient and dependent roles (Johnson, 1980, p. 137). The feminist theory also asserts that only men should commit sexual assault.

If the biosocial theory of sexual assault is correct, sexuality should have a great deal to do with the motivation behind sexual assaults, and both sexes (rather than just men) should be involved in committing such assaults. The theory also leads to the hypothesis that as the degree of physical force increases, the proportion of perpetrators who are men should become greater and greater. We can deduce the latter because the biosocial theory argues that, on average, (1) men's sex drives are stronger than women's and (2) men are less sensitive to pain (including pain inflicted on others) than are women.

This chapter assessed the merits of the biosocial theory by summarizing evidence that women do commit sexual assaults and that their contribution to these assaults gradually diminishes as the degree of physical force used increases. The overall findings from this meta-analysis support both theoretical hypotheses. First, while most studies of sexual assault have failed to ask men if they have been victimized or to ask women if they have been perpetrators, all of the exceptional studies have shown that not all sexual assaults are committed by men. Second, while many of the descriptions of the nature of sexual assaults by women against men were too vaguely described to be certain of their type, most of the evidence indicated that as the degree of physical force involved increases, the proportion of assaults by women dramatically decreases. The feminist theory is not capable of explaining what this analysis has documented.

The only evidence reviewed in this chapter that was contrary to the biosocial theory came from two studies that indicated that men were actually slightly more likely to be verbally coerced into having sex than were women. According to the biosocial theory, this should never happen because men's sex drive on average surpasses that of women. There may be ways of explaining the finding within the theory's framework. For example, it may partly reflect "wishful thinking" on the part of some men. In addition, women may be so much more accustomed to verbal pressure to have sex than men that instances in which women pressure men are more likely to be remembered.

Overall, the data summarized in Table 6.1 and Figure 6.2 are consistent with the biosocial theory and are impossible to explain from a feminist theoretical perspective. Most notably, the biosocial theory correctly predicted that women commit sexual assaults, albeit to a lesser degree than men. Furthermore, the theory correctly predicted that the proportion of male victims and female perpetrators would gradually decrease as the amount of physical force involved increased.

If the biosocial theory is correct, it is not true that sexual assaults are "pseudosexual acts." Rather, these assaults are an aspect of human sexuality that both sexes sometimes learn to exhibit. For a combination of evolutionary and neurohormonal reasons, the probability of men learning such behavior is much higher than it is for women, especially in the case of assaults involving the use of extreme physical force.

## REFERENCES

Anonymous. (1989, April). Offering resistance: How most people respond to rape. *Psychology Today, 23,* 13.

Bergada, I., & Bergada, C. (1995). Long term treatment with low dose testosterone in constitutional delay of growth and puberty: Effect on bone age maturation and pubertal progression. *Journal of Pediatric Endocrinology and Metabolism, 8,* 117–122.

Brownmiller, S. (1975). *Against our will: Men, women, and rape.* New York: Simon & Schuster.

Calderwood, D. (1987, May). The male rape victim. *Medical Aspects of Human Sexuality,* p. 53–55.

Chadwick, B. A., & Top, B. L. (1993). Religiosity and delinquency among LDS adolescents. *Journal for the Scientific Study of Religion, 32,* 51–67.

Dutton, D., & Painter, S. L. (1981). Traumatic bonding: The development of emotional attachments in battered women and other relationships of intermittent abuse. *Victimology, 6,* 139–155.

Eibl-Eibesfeldt, I. (1987). Ethological aspects of food sharing and the roots of possession. *South African Journal of Ethology, 10,* 23–28.

Ellis, L. (1989). *Theories of rape: Inquiries into the causes of sexual aggression.* New York: Hemisphere.

Ellis, L. (1991). A synthesized (biosocial) theory of rape. *Journal of Consulting and Clinical Psychology, 59,* 631–642.

Ellis, L. (1993). Rape as a biosocial phenomenon. In G. C. N. Hall, R. Hirschman, J. R. Graham, & M. S. Zaragoza (Eds.), *Sexual aggression: Issues in etiology, assessment, and treatment* (pp. 17–41). Washington, DC: Taylor & Francis.

Ellis, L., Hoffman, H., & Burke, D. M. (1990). Sex, sexual orientation, and criminal and violent behavior. *Personality and Individual Differences, 11,* 1207–1212.

Frazier, P. (1993). A comparative study of male and female rape victims seen at a hospital-based rape crisis program. *Journal of Interpersonal Violence, 8,* 64–76.

Groth, A. (1979). *Men who rape: The psychology of the offender.* New York: Plenum Press.

Groth, A., & Burgess, A. (1978). Rape: A pseudosexual act. *International Journal for Women's Studies, 1,* 207–210.

Groth, A., & Burgess, A. (1980). Male rape offenders and victims. *American Journal of Psychiatry, 137,* 806–810.

Hall, E., & Flannery, P. (1984). Prevalence and correlates of sexual assault experiences in adolescents. *Victimology: An International Journal, 9,* 398–406.

Halpern, C. T., Udry, J. R., Campbell, B., Suchindran, C., & Mason, G.

A. (1994). Testosterone and religiosity as predictors of sexual attitudes and activity among adolescent males: A biosocial model. *Journal of Biosocial Science, 26,* 217–234.

Hartless, J., Ditton, J., Nair, G., & Phillips, S. (1995). More sinned against than sinning. *British Journal of Criminology, 35,* 114–133.

Johnson, A. (1980). On the prevalence of rape in the United States. *Journal of Women in Culture and Society, 6,* 136–146.

Kanin, E. (1983). Rape as a function of relative sexual frustration. *Psychology Reports, 52,* 133–134.

Kanin, E. (1984). Date rape: Unofficial criminals and victims. *Victimology, 9,* 95–108.

Kaufman, A., Divasto, P., Jackson, R., Voorhees, D., & Christy, J. (1980). Male rape victims: Noninstitutionalized assault. *American Journal of Psychiatry, 137,* 221–223.

Kemper, T. (1990). *Social structure and testosterone.* New Brunswick, NJ: Rutgers University Press.

Kirkpatrick, C., & Kanin, E. (1957). Male sex aggression on a university campus. *American Sociological Review, 22,* 52–58.

Koskinen, S., & Martelin, T. (1994). Why are socioeconomic mortality differences smaller among women than among men? *Social Science and Medicine, 38,* 1385–1396.

Koss, M., Gidycz, C., & Wisniewski, N. (1987). The scope of rape: Incidence and prevalence of sexual aggression and victimization in a national sample of higher education students. *Journal of Consulting and Clinical Psychology, 55,* 162–170.

Koss, M., & Oros, C. (1982). Sexual Experiences Survey: A research instrument investigating sexual aggression and victimization. *Journal of Consulting and Clinical Psychology, 50,* 455–457.

Laumann, E., Gagnon, J., Michael, R., & Michaels, S. (1994). *The social organization of sexuality: Sexual practices in the United States.* Chicago: University of Chicago Press.

Lott, B., Reilly, M., & Howard, D. (1982). Sexual assault and harassment: A campus community case study. *Signs: Journal of Woman in Culture and Society, 8,* 296–319.

Low, B. S. (1990). Sex, power, and resources: Ecological correlates of sex differences. *International Journal of Contemporary Sociology, 27,* 50–73.

McConaghy, N. (1993). *Sexual behavior: Problems and management.* New York: Plenum Press.

Mills, J., Shiono, P., Shapiro, L., Crawford, P., & Rhoads, G. (1986). Early growth predicts timing of puberty in boys: Results of a 14-year nutrition and growth study. *Journal of Pediatrics, 109,* 543–547.

Moore, K., Nord, C., & Peterson, J. (1989). Nonvoluntary sexual activity among adolescents. *Family Planning Perspectives, 21,* 110–114.

Muehlenhard, C., & Cook, S. (1988). Men's self-reports of unwanted sexual activity. *Journal of Sex Research, 24,* 58–72.

Rouse, L. (1988). Abuse in dating relationships: A comparison of Blacks, Whites, and Hispanics. *Journal of College Student Development, 29,* 312–319.

Russell, D. (1984). *Sexual exploitation: Rape, child sexual abuse, and workplace harassment.* Beverly Hills, CA: Sage.

Sandberg, G., Jackson, T., & Petretic-Jackson, P. (1987). College students' attitudes regarding sexual coercion and aggression: Developing educational and preventive strategies. *Journal of College Student Personnel, 28,* 302–311.

Sattler, J. (1988). *Assessment of children's intelligence and other special abilities* (2nd ed.). Boston, MA: Allyn & Bacon.

Sigelman, C., Berry, C., & Wiles, K. (1984). Violence in college students' dating relationships. *Journal of Applied Social Psychology, 14,* 530–548.

Smith, M., & Bennett, N. (1985). Poverty, inequality, and theories of forcible rape. *Crime and Delinquency, 31,* 295–305.

Sorenson, S., & Siegel, J. (1992). Gender, ethnicity, and sexual assault: Findings from a Los Angeles study. *Journal of Social Issues, 48,* 93–104.

Sorenson, S., Stein, J., Siegel, J., Golding, J., & Burnam, M. (1987). Prevalence of adult sexual assault: The Los Angeles Epidemiologic Catchment Area Study. *American Journal of Epidemiology, 126,* 1154–1164.

Stets, J., & Pirog-Good, M. (1987). Violence in dating relationships. *Social Psychology Quarterly, 50,* 237–246.

Struckman-Johnson, C. (1988). Forced sex on dates: It happens to men, too. *The Journal of Sex Research, 24,* 234–241.

U.S. Department of Justice. (1989). *Sourcebook of criminal justice statistics, 1988.* Washington, DC: U.S. Government Printing Office.

# III

---

## COMPARISONS OF
## MALE AND
## FEMALE EXPERIENCES
## OF SEXUAL COERCION

This section is devoted to men's experiences with sexually aggressive women and how they compare to women's experiences with sexually aggressive men. In Chapter 7, Cindy Struckman-Johnson and David Struckman-Johnson present the results of their most recent survey of men who have experienced sexual coercion by women. They feature college men's verbatim descriptions of situations in which they felt pressured or forced to have sexual contact with a woman. The authors summarize their numerous investigations of the Sexual Opportunity Model—a framework for predicting when men will respond either favorably or negatively to a woman's coercive sexual advance.

This piece is followed by two critical analyses of the male and female experiences of sexual victimization in heterosexual relationships. In Chapter 8, prominent sex researchers E. Sandra Byers and Lucia F. O'Sullivan join in a superb review of the research on male and female victims of sexual coercion. They include data from their latest study of Canadian college students, conducted with their colleague Larry Finkelman. Readers will appreciate the authors' detailed summary table of the literature and their balanced discussion of the prevalence, context, and emotional impact of sexual coercion of men by women and women by men.

In Chapter 9, feminist researcher Wendy Stock presents a searing critique of research on sexual coercion of men by women. Stock argues that there is scant similarity between a man's typical encounter with female sexual coercion and a woman's typical encounter with male sexual coercion. Stock extends her analysis to recent popular books by Warren Farrell and Katie Roiphe, who downplay the severity of the problem of sexual coercion of women.

# 7

## The Dynamics and Impact
## of Sexual Coercion
## of Men by Women

CINDY STRUCKMAN-JOHNSON
DAVID STRUCKMAN-JOHNSON

"What happened to me occurred some years back on the east coast during my freshman year of college. I went to the beach one afternoon and was lying in a secluded section of dunes. Three young females discovered me, engaged me in a conversation, and after some brief dialogue, decided that they wanted, and were going to obtain, oral sex at my expense. One girl quickly pinned my arms back, the other grabbed my legs, while the third proceeded to pull my swimsuit down. She then began to masturbate me and then took my erection in her mouth. Initially I resisted, but as a young boy with 'active hormones' my resistance broke down, becoming a willing participant— caught up in the eroticism of the experience. The other two girls then took their turns (also oral sex). It was my first sexual encounter."

The description above was recently sent to us by a young man in a midwestern state who had read in a newspaper article that we studied sexual coercion of men. We have since corresponded several times with "Andrew" and have his permission to quote his story in this chapter. Whereas many people may think that Andrew's story is a freakish incident or perhaps a *Playboy* fantasy, we have learned in our research that Andrew is one of a substantial number of young men who have been coerced into sexual contact by sexually aggressive women. Many of these men, like Andrew, began to enjoy the sexual activity after initially resisting the advance. For other men, the experience was decidedly negative.

Our research on sexual coercion of men began in 1985, when we found that 16% of a sample of more than 200 men on our college campus had been forced to have sexual intercourse on a date during their lifetimes (Struckman-Johnson, 1988). We were taken aback by this outcome because we assumed that only women were sexually victimized in dating relationships. Although newspapers and magazines declared that we had made a startling "discovery," we were not the first researchers to document this phenomenon.

As early as 1984, Murphy found that 12% of men and 29% of women in a random sample of more than 400 students at a Minnesota university had succumbed to "forced intercourse on a date" (see Murphy, 1988). In 1987, Sandberg, Jackson, and Petretic-Jackson reported that 25% of men and 48% of women, out of more than 400 students surveyed in classrooms at a South Dakota university, had been "sexually assaulted" (touched, held, or kissed against their will) by a dating partner.

In that same year, two large-scale studies involving representative sampling of several thousand adults revealed that men in urban community settings were victims of sexual coercion. Sorenson, Stein, Siegel, Golding, and Burnam (1987) estimated that 7% of men and 13% of women in the Los Angeles area had been pressured or forced to have sexual contact since the age of 16. Among white men aged 18–39 years, the assault rate was 16%. Approximately 70% of the assaults were carried out by a woman (Struckman-Johnson, 1991). A second survey (Cameron, Proctor, Cameron, Coburn, & Forde, 1987) found that 6% of men and 22% of women between the ages of 18 and 25 years living in Denver, Los Angeles, District of Columbia, Louisville, and Omaha had been forced into sexual activity against their will. Approximately one-half of the male victims said they had been "raped" by a woman.

In 1988, the year that our first study was published, several other researchers presented similar findings. Aizenman and Kelley (1988) reported that 14% of men and 29% of women in a random sample of more than 300 New Jersey college students had been forced to have intercourse against their will. Poppen and Segal (1988) found that 18% of men and 37% of women in a small representative sample of students at a Washington, DC, university had been coerced into having sexual intercourse. Also that year, Muehlenhard and Cook (1988) published their now-famous study showing that 24% of men and 32% of women from a classroom sample of nearly 1,000 Texas college students engaged in unwanted sexual activity due to physical coercion or restraint.

Although we expected that research on sexual coercion of men by women would surge in the 1990s, only a small number of studies have addressed this topic to date. In 1991, Lottes found that 24% of the men and 35% of the women in a representative classroom sample of more than 300 Maryland university students had been coerced into sexual intercourse. Men indicated that women used nonphysical tactics of verbal pressure, deceitful statements, or intoxication to have sex with them. In 1993, Anderson and Aymami published a significant work revealing that women used a wide variety of strategies to initiate sex with men. According to their classroom survey of students at a New York university, 16% of 128 men reported that a woman had used physical force in an attempt to initiate sex with them.

Also in 1993, Benson Hoffman, an undergraduate at Antioch College, Ohio, conducted an interesting unpublished study of sexual coercion of men for his senior honors thesis. Hoffman's research is especially notable because it occurred the year that Antioch adopted a sexual offense policy that required students to ask for verbal consent to initiate sexual contact ("Sober Orgies Only," 1993). Hoffman distributed surveys to 161 men living in a residence hall and received 68 back. Forty percent of the men reported coercive sexual contact and 27% had experienced coercive sexual intercourse with a woman since the age of 16. Women were most likely to use verbal persuasion and intoxication to initiate sex. However, men described aggressive advances in which they were "jumped" on during study sessions, pushed up against walls and cars, forcefully kissed in public places, mounted while sleeping in their beds, and pressured out of their rooms by a woman who refused to leave. At least one man reported that at age 16, he was physically held down and raped by his roommate's female friend.

In the mid-1990s, several well-known magazines commissioned surveys which included questions on forced sex. For example, *Esquire* magazine (Goodman, 1994) reported that 29% of 1,000 women aged 18–25 years responded that they had pressured a man into having sex. According to a *Details magazine* survey of readers aged 18–34 years ("Love Rules," 1994), 18% of female respondents indicated that they had coerced someone into having sex.

At least one survey published in 1994 suggested that sexual coercion of men occurs infrequently. In their landmark study, *The Social Organization of Sexuality,* Laumann, Gagnon, Michael, and Michaels (1994) found that only 1.5% of men as compared to 22% of women from a national sample of 3,000 respondents reported that a member of the opposite gender had forced them to do something sexual. The authors did not present the male data by age group, so the forced-sex rate for young men is not known. It should be noted that the rate for women was based upon an anonymous survey and interview data, whereas the men's rate reflected only interview data.

In 1996, Lavoie and Poitras published an important survey of coercive sexuality among a classroom sample of more than 600 adolescents in Quebec, Canada. Their results showed that 10% of boys and 24% of girls with heterosexual dating experience sustained unwanted intercourse due to coercive tactics, which included verbal coercion, misuse of authority, alcohol, and physical force. Both girls and boys reported that, in most cases, their partners used verbal coercion to obtain sexual contact. This study is one of the first to document that both sexes sustain coercive sexual experiences in high school dating.

Young men in other countries may also experience sexual aggression, although perhaps not to the same degree as American men. Lottes and Weinberg (1996) discovered that 22% of a sample of young Swedish men, as compared to 50% of an American sample of men, reported being subjected to nonphysical sexual coercion by a woman.

In summary, the literature indicates that between the ages of 16 and 40 years, as few as 1% to as many as 50% of boys and men may experience sexually coercive contact with a woman. The goal of our research for the past 10 years has been to understand the dynamics and emotional impact of these coercive incidents.

First, we have asked questions about men's relationships with sexually aggressive women. For example, is the advance typically made by a girlfriend who is being innovative in her sexual approach or is it made by a bold (or desperate) stranger trying to get a man's attention? Second, we have examined the tactics women use to get sex from reluctant men. For example, how can women "talk" men into having sex? How can a woman engineer sex with a thoroughly intoxicated man or physically restrain a larger, stronger man?

Finally, we have tried to discover how men feel about coercive sexual advances. In our original study, men's reactions ranged from good to neutral to bad. Other research has also documented men's ambivalent reactions. Long and Muehlenhard (1987) found that college men had a mixture of negative (sad, uncomfortable) and positive (feeling cared for, confident of manhood) reactions to unwanted sexual contact. According to Siegel, Golding, Stein, Burnam, and Sorenson (1990), only one-fourth to one-third of men who were sexually assaulted reported significant emotional reactions. Such results have led us to ask what makes men upset with a coercive advance—is it the type of woman, the tactics she uses, or the level of sexual activity that results?

We have found tentative answers to many of our questions by asking college men to tell us what happened during their actual experiences with sexually aggressive women. In 1990, 5 years following our original survey (Struckman-Johnson, 1988), we conducted a second study of several hundred men in psychology classes at the University of South Dakota (Struckman-Johnson & Struckman-Johnson, 1994a). Instead of asking about "forced sexual intercourse," we refined our approach and asked men if they had ever been "pressured or forced" to engage in sexual touching or intercourse (Sorenson et al., 1987). Participants then gave additional information about the most recent incident. We asked respondents about same-sex, as well as opposite-sex, experiences.

We found that 30% of men had had at least one coercive experience with a woman since the age of 16. The incident involved sexual touch for 23% and intercourse for 20% of the men. A majority of men were verbally pressured into sexual contact. Only 12% of the men (less than 1% of the sample) had a force tactic used against them. Most men were not very upset by the incident—only one-fifth reported strong negative reactions. Overall, men with and without coercion experience (regardless of initiator gender) did not differ on measures of sexual self-esteem.

In 1995, we conducted a third survey (Struckman-Johnson, 1995) to obtain a 10-year update on the incidence and dynamics of sexual coercion of men on our campus. We used the same instrument and procedures developed in our 1990 study but restricted questions to experiences with women. The methods and results are described in the following sections.

## METHOD

### Participants

Participants were 318 men enrolled in psychology courses at the University of South Dakota in the 1994–1995 academic year. A majority of respondents were Caucasian with middle-class backgrounds. After we excluded four men who did not complete the survey, the final sample consisted of 314 men aged 18–45 years (mean = 20.8).

### Instrument

To assess coercive touch, participants were asked: "Since the age of 16, have you ever been pressured or forced by a girl or woman to have sexual contact which involved touching of sexual parts of your body (but not intercourse)?" For intercourse, the question read: "Since the age of 16, have you ever been pressured or forced by a girl or a woman to have sexual contact which involved having sexual intercourse?" Respondents were asked how many times these events had happened.

Participants then answered questions about the *most recent episode* of sexual touch or intercourse, which included initiator relationship, the kind of pressure or force used, and the sexual acts that occurred. They were asked to give a brief description of what happened and to explain the person's motives. Finally, participants rated the "extent that this event has had a negative impact upon you." The scale ranged from 1 ("has had no negative effect upon me") to 7 ("has had a severe negative effect upon me").

## Procedures

The researcher invited male students in general psychology, social psychology, sex roles, and sexuality classes to take a short anonymous survey about coercive sexual experiences for extra credit points. Interested men were instructed to take a survey and a consent form to complete in the privacy of their homes. The following class period, students turned in the surveys and signed consent forms in separate collection boxes. Over 90% of men in the classes participated.

## RESULTS

### Incidence Rates

As shown in Table 7.1, 43% of the men reported having had at least one coercive sexual experience with a woman since the age of 16. Thirty-six percent of the men had had at least one incident of sexual touch. Half of this group said that they had only been touched once, but the other half reported from 2 to 30 incidents. On the average, men with sexual touch experience reported 2.3 incidents. Twenty-seven percent of the men reported at least one incident involving intercourse. Of this group, a little over half said that it had only happened once, but the others reported from 2 to 15 incidents. On the average, men reporting intercourse incidents had experienced 1.4 events.

TABLE 7.1. Male Participants by Experience of Coercive Sexual Touch and Intercourse

| Type of coercion | Participants | |
|---|---|---|
| | N | % |
| No coercive intercourse or coercive touch | 180 | 57 |
| Coercive touch but no coercive intercourse | 51 | 16 |
| Coercive intercourse but no coercive touch | 22 | 7 |
| Coercive intercourse and coercive touch | 61 | 20 |
| Total | 314 | 100 |

## Initiator Relationship and Strategy

Fifty-one men gave information about a sexual touch incident, and 83 men described an intercourse incident. As shown in Table 7.2, over half of all incidents occurred with an acquaintance/friend/new date, about one-third occurred with a girlfriend/fiancée, and less than 10% were committed by a stranger. Intercourse incidents were more likely than touch incidents to involve girlfriends/fiancées, whereas touch incidents were somewhat more likely than intercourse incidents to involve strangers.

Three-fourths of coerced men were pressured by persuasion (Table 7.3). The second most common tactic was "got you drunk"—reported by 40% of coerced men. The third most common strategy was threat of love withdrawal—cited by about 19% of men. Physical restraint was reported in only 8% of the incidents. Only one man reported being physically harmed. The strategies used in touch and intercourse incidents were relatively similar, except that intoxication was reported more frequently among intercourse incidents.

We conducted further analyses to find that 90% of all incidents involved only pressure tactics (persuasion, bribe, love withdrawal, and intoxication). Persuasion was the sole tactic used in 43% of the cases. In another 16% of the cases, the tactics of persuasion and intoxication were used together. Only 10% of the incidents involved at least one force tactic (fear, threatened harm, physical restraint, physical harm, weapon). Physical restraint was the most common force tactic reported.

TABLE 7.2. Relationship of Female Initiator to Male Receiver

| Relationship | Sexual touch | | Sexual intercourse | | Overall | |
|---|---|---|---|---|---|---|
| | N | % | N | % | N | % |
| Stranger | 7 | 14 | 3 | 4 | 10 | 7 |
| Acquaintance, friend, new date | 32 | 63 | 42 | 50 | 74 | 56 |
| Girlfriend, fiancée | 9 | 17 | 34 | 41 | 43 | 32 |
| Spouse, ex-spouse | 1 | 2 | 1 | 1 | 2 | 1 |
| Relative | 0 | 0 | 0 | 0 | 0 | 0 |
| Other (e.g., employer) | 2 | 4 | 3 | 4 | 5 | 4 |
| Total | 51 | 100 | 83 | 100 | 134 | 100 |

TABLE 7.3. Strategy Used by Female Initiator

| Strategy | Sexual touch (total N = 51) | | Sexual intercourse (total N = 83) | | Overall (total N = 134) | |
|---|---|---|---|---|---|---|
| | N | % | N | % | N | % |
| Persuasion | 41 | 80 | 59 | 71 | 100 | 75 |
| Bribe | 3 | 6 | 5 | 6 | 8 | 6 |
| Love withdrawal | 6 | 12 | 19 | 23 | 25 | 19 |
| Got you drunk | 15 | 29 | 39 | 47 | 54 | 40 |
| Scared you because they were bigger and stronger | 0 | 0 | 0 | 0 | 0 | 0 |
| Threaten harm | 1 | 2 | 1 | 1 | 2 | 1 |
| Physical restraint | 5 | 10 | 6 | 7 | 11 | 8 |
| Physically harmed you | 0 | 0 | 1 | 1 | 1 | 1 |
| Weapon present | 0 | 0 | 0 | 0 | 0 | 0 |

*Note.* Column *N*'s sum to greater than total *N* and column percentages sum to more than 100 because of multiple strategies used in some incidents.

## Descriptions of Touch Incidents

The men who described a sexual-touch incident revealed that, in most cases, a female acquaintance touched them in an unsuccessful bid to have sexual intercourse. The men prevented further activity by saying no or leaving the situation. From these descriptions, we learned that many men consider oral sex to be "touching," although we included oral sex in our definition of intercourse in the survey. We also learned that "penis grabbing" is a major female technique of initiating sex, although generally ineffective in these cases.

We chose the following responses to illustrate the variety of coercive touch situations that men encountered. The original grammar and spelling are preserved. Some men were surprised but not upset by the sexual fondling of acquaintances who unexpectedly showed their attraction to them. The following is a description of how one man tolerated the persistent advance of an acquaintance:

"Sitting on couch together watching tv. She leans over and kissed me by surprise and grabbed my penis. She wanted to have sex but I said no because I have a girlfriend. She said she didn't care and then proceeded to give me a blowjob through my pants while unzipping them. I stopped her and she understood. She still tries when we are alone but so far my morals have held out (whew!)."

Another man said he was pleased but too shocked to pursue sex with an acquaintance who made the following advance:

"We were playing basketball in my backyard one summer night. The ball went back into the grove and so I went to get it. She came up from behind me, threw me on the grass and laid on me and kissed me. She put my hands on her breasts and started taking our clothes off. She proceeded with oral sex and when she was about to initiate intercourse our friends pulled into the driveway."

A more typical situation was one in which the man was *not* pleased with the pursuit of a female acquaintance. One wrote:

"The woman after getting drunk showed up at my door came in and proceed to undress herself and started to remove my clothes. She performed fellatio on me and ask me to have intercourse. I told her no. She asked why not. I stated that I didn't want her to use me and to leave."

In the following two descriptions, the men indicated that they were intoxicated and that the female acquaintance used physical restraint in her attempt to have sex:

"When I was about 16, I was at a friend's house. She wanted my help getting a box out of her room. When I got up there she grabbed my hand & before I knew it my hand was on her breast. I pulled away and she yanked my other hand to do the same thing. I stopped her again. Then she grabbed at the penis. I pulled away & yelled or asked her what she was doing this for. Turned out that she thought the feelings were the same for me."

"I went up to go to the bathroom and she followed me upstairs and I was then hiding and she forced me on the bed and started kissing me but I didn't kiss her and then I tried getting up but she pushed me back down but then I just threw her off me and ran down the stairs."

Several men described incidents in which a new date tried to initiate sexual contact at a time when the men were not prepared for it. In one case, a man broke up with a "mental" woman who repeatedly pressured for sex in their first weeks of dating. In the following example, the man described how a new date used a tactic of "persuasion" to attempt first-time sex:

"We dated a couple of times before anything happened. We were alone in the house and she pulled me into the back bedroom (not rough like). She undressed me and kept touching me. I was scared, and didn't really know what to do. I told her so, and that I want to leave. She got undressed while holding me down (again not really very rough, I probably could have gotten up). That really scared me and then she let me up knowing for sure that I felt uneasy. I got dressed and left. We were friends for a long time after that but it wasn't the same."

Some of the men were sexually touched by uninhibited female strangers in bars. One man was quite offended when an unknown woman started to touch his genitals under the table. Another said that a woman came up and grabbed his penis in order to win a bet with her friends. One man wrote:

"The young lady just starting kissing me and grabbing my dick. Because I was drunk and didn't know the girl I do kind of wish it wouldn't have happened. I'm glad I didn't go all the way with her."

Men were also likely to be touched by strangers at house parties:

"I was drunk at a party and a large girl kept trying to kiss me and put her hands down my pants. I kept backing off but she became more persistent so I took off and stayed close to my friends so she wouldn't bug me anymore."

## Descriptions of Intercourse Incidents

We found that the intercourse responses revealed more complicated situations than the touch incidents. Most of the intercourse incidents initiated by an acquaintance/friend/new date (about half of all intercourse incidents) could best be described as a "one-night stand." In a typical scenario, a man (usually intoxicated) was pressured to have sex with a woman (often intoxicated) whom he was not romantically involved with. Many of the episodes started at bars, such as this incident brought about by persuasion and intoxication:

> "While working in California, some friends and I frequented a particular dance club on weekends. One Friday after a twelve hour shift, I was at the club till closing and a young lady I had met there offered me a ride home. Between lack of sleep and excess alcohol I took leave of my senses and was persuaded into sexual intercourse."

The following case also resulted from persuasion and alcohol. The man was particularly upset because, in retrospect, he felt the woman was trying to break up his engagement:

> "I went to a bar with some girls from work. We all got very drunk and while at the bar both girls started kissing on me and claiming they wanted to be with me. While I found this all flattering I had no intentions of having sex with either one. Once the bar closed I had to give one of the girls a ride home, when we got to her apt. she invited me in. I did not refuse her offer but was still not intending on having sex. However she was. Once inside the apt. she (wasting no time) forced herself on me, began oral sex and ultimately intercourse took place."

Undesired one-night stands were likely to happen at house parties that combined easy access to alcohol and bedrooms. All of the following cases involved a female acquaintance who used persuasion and intoxication:

> "I was at a party, & sitting in this room by my self. The girl who owned the house came in & locked the door. She then got on top of me & started kissing me. I was very intoxicated, & she convinced me to sex with her."

> "I was in bed after a night of drinking and an intoxicated girl acquaintance of mine came in my room and came on to me. At

first I request her to leave because she wasn't very attractive, she persisted and I gave in and had intercourse. . . . She was attracted to me and knew I wouldn't do anything unless I was drunk."

Some men were so intoxicated that a female acquaintance was able to have sex with them without the consent or active participation of the man. In the following incidents, the woman was an acquaintance, and the tactic was marked as intoxication. Some of these descriptions help explain the mechanics of how women can achieve sex with intoxicated men:

"We were at her friends house and were drinking cherry vodka. I was very drunk very fast. She took me to the bathroom and I ended up on the bathroom floor. She took off my pants and engaged in oral intercourse on me. That's all I remember."

"Intercourse did not totally occur. I was drunk and we were making out. We both were naked and she just sat down on my penis. When I realized what she was doing I pushed her off and stopped making out."

"I was at prom and got drunk. I passed out/fell asleep on a bed. She grabbed my penis and started to have oral sex. When I became erect she took her clothes off and tried to have intercourse with me but I stopped her."

In most incidents, the tactic of "intoxication" ("got you drunk") was actually a case where the men themselves became drunk or were drinking with others. However, in the incident below, the man viewed the woman as intentionally getting him drunk:

"This girl who I was at a party talking to offer me drink after drink. Once alone with her and 'making out' she pulled down my pants and hers and put my erection in her vagina. She had sex with me for about 5 minutes when a friend saved me & came into the room and helped me get away."

In the following situations, the men indicated that a female acquaintance used physical restraint:

"She was all over me. She was grabbing me and licking me. She got on top of me and just pushed it in as she held me down."

"She got me drunk and tied me up and then had sex with me 6 times in 1 night. She was an ex-girlfriend and was getting back at me for dumping her. She was psycho."

Another type of intercourse incident was one in which a man felt he could not say no to the advance of a female acquaintance because of standards of masculinity. This situation is illustrated by the following two incidents in which the woman used persuasion:

"It was in high school and the girl I was with had just broken up with her steady boyfriend. We met at a party and she came on to me. She sat down to talk and I asked her what she like to do for fun and she said 'fuck.' I couldn't believe she would say that then she took it to that extreme. I felt that if I didn't she would tell everyone I was a loser."

"Me and a friend went out and we ended making out. She wanted to have intercourse but I didn't feel that attracted to her at the time. I ended up having sex just because she was so persistent and I didn't want to feel like a wimp."

A few men were persuaded to have sex with acquaintances because they became physically aroused. This man's description reveals the mixed feelings of a man confronted with an unexpected sexual advance from someone he did not know well:

"She entered my dorm room while I was alone and asked if I liked surprises. I said sure, so she told me to close me eyes she then grabbed my genital area and began kissing me. I asked what she was doing and she said she didn't know and didn't care. I was uncomfortable at first but then began to enjoy her. She then revealed a condom and asked me to have sex with her. I regretfully did."

An entirely different set of dynamics happened when men were with girlfriends. In these situations, the men most likely had an ongoing sexual relationship with the woman that made her advance less surprising and more acceptable. In some instances, a girlfriend's coercive advance could best be described as a sex game of "mock force." For example, some men said that their girlfriends playfully forced them into intercourse as a way of spicing up their sex lives. Most (but not all) men in this situation were pleased with the advance.

In other situations, men said that their girlfriends were sexually aroused and demanded immediate gratification. Although not in the mood, the men dutifully and often resentfully engaged in intercourse. In one unusual case, a man indicated that he was physically harmed by his girlfriend when he said no:

"I visited my girlfriend after drinking w/guy friends. She was horny and I wasn't. We had sex once, but I was hit and yelled at when I wanted to leave w/out doing it again. I made her happy, waited for her to fall asleep/pass out, and left."

Another notable type of incident was when girlfriends pressured sexually inexperienced men into intercourse at a time when the men did not want to lose their virginity. One wrote:

"She got me drunk & persuaded me. I had told her previously that I didn't want to have sex until I was married. She apologized the next day."

Very few intercourse incidents happened with strangers or persons in "other" relationships, such as an employer. However, two cases stood out. One man in his forties recalled a situation in which he was being interviewed by a reporter. She promised him she would write his biography and invited him to her apartment to continue the interview. She then told him she would not write about him unless he had sex with her. The second case was another variation of blackmail. Although we have received a few reports of male and female students having sex with teachers in previous studies, this situation added a new twist:

"A teacher in high school found out I slept with a different teacher. She threatened to expose the situation if I didn't sleep with her."

# Perceived Motivation
# of Initiator

The men were asked to explain, "What do you think was the person's motive for doing this?" A content analysis of answers revealed that 38% of the men attributed the woman's advance to sexual arousal and "horniness." Other common attributions were liking and love for the man (16%), loneliness and need for intimacy (10%), and alcohol effects (9%).

## Negative Impact of Incidents

On the average, men rated the negative impact of the incident at 3.0 on a 7-point scale. The score indicated that men were only mildly upset by a typical incident. One-third of the men gave the incident a 1 rating—indicating there was no negative impact. Nearly 30% gave the incident a 2 to 3 rating, suggesting that some negative impact occurred. About 23% rated the incident in the 4 to 5 range, indicating that they were moderately upset. Another 14% experienced severe negative impact, as reflected by ratings of 6 to 7.

We conducted an analysis to explore what factors may be related to greater negative impact of incidents. Unfortunately, the number of incidents involving force was too small ($N = 14$) to compare with those involving pressure. As an alternative, we compared the effects of having a romantic relationship with the initiator (girlfriend/fiancées vs. others), sexual outcome (touch vs. intercourse), and use of the intoxication strategy. We predicted that advances of nonromantic women and acts involving intoxication would have a greater negative impact. We also expected that acts of intercourse with nonromantic women under conditions of intoxication would be associated with high negative impact.

A 2 (relationship) by 2 (sexual outcome) by 2 (intoxication) analysis of variance of impact scores revealed only a significant effect for intoxication, $F(7, 124) = 18.05$; $p < .04$. As expected, men who marked the "got you drunk" tactic rated the incident as having a higher negative impact (mean = 3.44, $N = 54$) than did men who did not (mean = 2.7, $N = 78$).

# DISCUSSION

In summary, 43% of a sample of 314 college men reported having had a sexually coercive experience with a woman since the age of 16. The 1995 rate is higher than the 30% rate found in our 1990 survey, which used similar procedures. The disparity in rates may reflect differences in the characteristics of the two samples. Or it may indicate that women's sexually aggressive behavior increased over the 5-year period.

The majority of the most recent incidents were initiated by a female acquaintance who used pressure tactics (most likely persuasion and intoxication). Our results suggest that intoxication may be the "great equalizer" when it comes to men's and women's vulnerability to sexual exploitation. Women's use of physical coercion was low—only 14 men (10% of the coerced sample and 0.05% of the sample) had a force tactic used against them. A majority of the most recent incidents resulted in the act of sexual intercourse.

As found in our 1990 study (Struckman-Johnson & Struckman-Johnson, 1994a), the emotional impact of the incident varied considerably. One-third of the men were not upset at all, about one-third were mildly upset, and more than a third were moderately to extremely upset by the incident. However, explaining why men had these reactions has been a challenge. It is difficult to compare men's reactions to real-life incidents reported in survey data because each man's incident occurred in unique circumstances. In addition, the sample sizes of some incident categories (i.e., use of force tactics, stranger initiators) have been too small to conduct statistically reliable comparisons.

Therefore, we have supplemented our survey data by conducting studies on how men *think* they would react if they were the target of a woman's forceful sexual advance. We have presented men with written scenarios describing how a woman comes to their room and initiates a sexual act—usually by physically pushing or holding the man down and touching his genitals. The men estimate their reactions to this situation, including the degree of negative impact of the incident. By experimentally varying qualities of the initiator, the tactics used, and the sexual act attempted, we have determined men's anticipated reactions to a wide variety of sexual advance situations.

Based on our vignette and survey research, we have developed the Sexual Opportunity Model to explain why men experience a range of positive to negative reactions to coercive sexual contact with women (Struckman-Johnson & Struckman-Johnson, 1996). We propose that because young men value and enjoy sex, they are predisposed to view a woman's aggressive advance as a positive sexual opportunity, not a violation of will (Smith, Pine, & Hawley, 1988). The average man is likely to interpret the woman's advance as an act of sexual seduction, not aggression. Freed from the risks and responsibility of initiating sex, a man has the option of enjoying sex with a woman who unequivocally desires him.

However, a man's reaction to the advance is mediated by at least four factors: (1) the degree to which the advance violates his personal sexual standards; (2) the level of force used by the woman; (3) the degree to which the woman is sexually desirable or creates sexual arousal by her actions; and (4) the extent to which a romantic relationship with the woman justifies the act. Men will respond favorably when conditions are optimal for viewing the advance as a sexual opportunity—low violation of standards, low coercion, high sexual desirability, and high level of romantic relationship with the initiator. To the extent that these conditions are not met, men will tend to respond negatively.

To date, the results of our vignette and survey research largely support the Sexual Opportunity Model. Our strongest findings are summarized below:

1. *Men tend to respond positively to a forceful sexual advance from a woman with whom they have a romantic/sexual relationship.* Based on a vignette study, we have learned that a majority of men are pleased by the idea of a physically forceful advance initiated by a steady girlfriend with whom they have already had sex. Men interpret this situation as a sexual game in which their partner is using force to seduce them. They view the use of force as either play behavior or as an indication of the woman's intense sexual desire for them. In either case, they welcome the advance as a change from the routine in which men are in charge of initiating sex (Struckman-Johnson & Struckman-Johnson, 1996).

Our survey research has been less clear on the relationship factor. In the 1995 survey, there was no difference in the negative impact of incidents initiated by romantic partners versus others. However, we have noted that in all three surveys, many men who were forcefully seduced by girlfriends commented that they actually enjoyed the experience.

2. *Men tend to respond positively to a forceful sexual advance from a very attractive woman.* Based on a vignette study, a majority of men report that they would be pleased to have a sexually desirable woman physically force them to have sex, even if she is only an acquaintance. Many men have told us that it is one of their sexual fantasies to be forcefully taken by an attractive woman. They interpret her use of force not as dangerous aggression but as a show of strong sexual desire (Struckman-Johnson & Struckman-Johnson, 1994b). We do not have evidence from our survey data to support the "beauty bias" effect because we have not yet asked men to describe the appearance of the initiator.

3. *Men tend to respond negatively to a forceful sexual advance when the women threatens or demonstrates capacity to harm.* According to our vignette research, men are somewhat tolerant of the idea of being physically restrained by a woman who is trying to have sex with them. We speculate that men are not very upset by being held down because (a) they view the action as playful restraint or (b) they assume that they can use their strength to stop her. However, if the vignette woman is said to hold the man down *and* threatens to hurt him or carries a weapon, a majority of men say that they will be moderately upset. They would perceive her as dangerous and perhaps mentally disturbed (Struckman-Johnson & Struckman-Johnson, 1994b).

Data from all three surveys have generally supported the force effect. Although only small numbers of men have reported that force tactics were used against them, most of these men indicated that the incident had a moderate to severe negative impact.

4. *Men tend to respond negatively to the forceful sexual advance of a female stranger.* Based upon our vignette research, a majority of men say they will reject the advance of a woman who is described as a relative stranger—someone they have known only a few hours. They would distrust her motives, view her as having mental problems or nymphomania, as being desperate, or as likely to have a venereal disease (Struckman-Johnson & Struckman-Johnson, 1996). We do not have evidence of this effect in our survey data because so few incidents were perpetrated by strangers.

5. *Men tend to respond negatively to a forceful sexual advance of an unattractive woman regardless of force level used.* Our vignette research

has revealed that men have strong negative reactions to the imagined advance of an unattractive woman. Approximately 90% of men said they would not have sex with a very unattractive woman, even if she approached them with a gentle touch. Apparently men feel that unattractive women are sexually undesirable and socially unacceptable as sex partners (Struckman-Johnson & Struckman-Johnson, 1994b). We have some corroboration from our survey data in that numerous men have reported being upset by advances from women described as unattractive, large, fat, and "beyond my acceptable weight limit."

6. *Men tend to respond negatively to a woman's forceful sexual advance if it is contrary to their beliefs about casual sex, losing their virginity, or being faithful to a romantic partner.* Our research consistently indicates that many men have high standards of sexual conduct that can be violated by a woman's forceful advance. In a recent vignette study, we found that men who had more restricted sexual standards as measured by the Sociosexual Orientation Inventory (Simpson & Gangestad, 1991) had a significantly more negative reaction to a coercive sexual advance by a woman than did men with less restricted sexual standards. In the same study, men who were told to assume that they had a serious girlfriend had a more negative reaction to the vignette woman than did men who assumed that they were available for a relationship (Struckman-Johnson & Struckman-Johnson, 1997).

In our survey research, we have identified at least two standards that are threatened by women's advances. First, we have found many cases where men deeply regretted losing their virginity to the wrong woman or at the wrong time in their lives. In many cases, the men were dating "older women" in high school who pressured them into sex. Second, men reported being very upset when an acquaintance or an ex-girlfriend initiated sex with them, resulting in betrayal of their current romantic partner.

7. *Men tend to respond negatively if a woman takes advantage of their intoxicated state to have sex with them.* We tested the intoxication factor in our 1995 survey because we noted that numerous men were very upset by having a drunken one-night stand with an unfamiliar woman. The results suggest that men do not like anyone to sexually exploit them while they are intoxicated. We will have to adjust the Sexual Opportunity Model to include a condition for men's perceived level of control in responding to the advance.

In conclusion, our research shows that men's reactions to women's sexual coercion are clearly influenced by qualities of the woman, the tactics used, and men's personal values. In future research, we would like to determine if men perceive women to be truly capable of physically forcing a man to have sex. We speculate that one major sex difference in response to sexual coercion is that women fear that they can be overpowered, but men assume that they can control or escape the situation. We would also like to investigate whether men who report high negative impact from a sexual coercion incident have subsequent sexual, psychological, or relationship problems.

Finally, we plan to continue work on the Sexual Opportunity Model, with particular emphasis on men's sexual standards. Eventually, we hope that our research will help dispel some of the old negative stereotypes that portray men as "sexual predators." In contrast, our research consistently indicates that men do not leap at every sexual opportunity, that they are guided by sexual standards, and that they are indeed vulnerable to the sexual aggression of women.

## REFERENCES

Aizenman, M., & Kelley, G. (1988). The incidence of violence and acquaintance rape in dating relationships among college men and women. *Journal of College Student Development, 29,* 305–311.

Anderson, P., & Aymami, R. (1993). Reports of female initiation of sexual contact: Male and female differences. *Archives of Sexual Behavior, 22*(4), 335–343.

Cameron, P., Proctor, K., Cameron, K., Coburn, W., & Forde, N. (1987). *Is the rape rate increasing?* Paper presented at the annual meeting of the Eastern Psychological Association, Washington, DC.

Goodman, E. (1994, February). Would one thousand young American women . . . ? *Esquire, 121,* 65–67.

Hoffman, B. (1993). *Men at Antioch College: Pressured and forced sexual experience.* Unpublished manuscript, Antioch College.

Laumann, E., Gagnon, J., Michael, R., & Michaels, S. (1994). *The social organization of sexuality: Sexual practices in the United States.* Chicago: University of Chicago Press.

Lavoie, F., & Poitras, M. (1996). A study of the prevalence of sexual coercion in adolescent dating relationships in a Quebec sample. *Victims and Violence, 10,* 125–139.

Long, P., & Muehlenhard, C. (1987, April). *Why some men don't say no: A comparison of men who did versus did not resist pressure to have unwanted sexual intercourse.* Paper presented at the midcontinent meeting of the Society for the Scientific Study of Sex, Bloomington, IN.

Lottes, I. (1991). The relationship between nontraditional gender roles and sexual coercion. *Journal of Psychology and Human Sexuality, 4*(4), 89–109.

Lottes, I., & Weinberg, M. (1996). Sexual coercion among university students: A comparison of the United States and Sweden. *Journal of Sex Research, 34,* 67–76.

Love rules: The 1994 *Details* survey on romance and the state of our union. (1994, May). *Details, 12,* 108–113.

Muehlenhard, C., & Cook, S. (1988). Men's self-reports of unwanted sexual activity. *Journal of Sex Research, 24,* 58–72.

Murphy, J. (1988). Date abuse and forced intercourse among college students. In G. P. Hotaling, D. Finkelhor, J. T. Kirkpatrick, & M. A. Straus (Eds.), *Family abuse and its consequences: New directions in research* (pp. 285–296). Beverly Hills, CA: Sage.

Poppen, P., & Segal, N. (1988). The influence of sex and sex role orientation on sexual coercion. *Sex Roles, 19,* 689–701.

Sandberg, G., Jackson, T., & Petretic-Jackson, P. (1987). College dating attitudes regarding sexual coercion and sexual aggression: Developing education and prevention strategies. *Journal of College Student Personnel, 28,* 302–310.

Siegel, J., Golding, J., Stein, J., Burnam, M., & Sorenson, S. (1990). Reactions to sexual assault: A community study. *Journal of Interpersonal Violence, 5,* 229–246.

Simpson, J. A., & Gangestad, S. W. (1991). Individual differences in sociosexuality: Evidence for convergent and discriminant validity. *Journal of Personality and Social Psychology, 60,* 870–883.

Smith, R., Pine, C., & Hawley, M. (1988). Social cognition about adult male victims of female sexual assault. *Journal of Sex Research, 24,* 101–112.

Sober orgies only. (1993, October 11). *Time, 142,* 24.

Sorenson, S., Stein, J., Siegel, J., Golding, J., & Burnam, M. (1987). The prevalence of adult sexual assault: The Los Angeles Epidemiologic Catchment Area Project. *American Journal of Epidemiology, 126,* 1154–1164.

Struckman-Johnson, C. (1988). Forced sex on dates: It happens to men, too. *Journal of Sex Research, 24,* 234–241.

Struckman-Johnson, C. (1991). Male victims of acquaintance rape. In A. Parrot and L. Bechhofer (Eds.), *Acquaintance rape: The hidden crime* (pp. 192–214). New York: Wiley.

Struckman-Johnson, C. (1995, November). The dynamics and impact of women's sexual coercion of college men. In C. Muehlenhard (Chair), *Sexual coercion of men by women: Implications for the role of gender and the role of politics in sexual science.* Symposium conducted at the annual meeting of the Society for the Scientific Study of Sex, San Francisco, CA.

Struckman-Johnson, C., & Struckman-Johnson, D. (1994a). Men pressured and forced into sexual experience. *Archives of Sexual Behavior, 23,* 93–114.

Struckman-Johnson, C., & Struckman-Johnson, D. (1994b). Men's reactions to hypothetical sexual advances: A beauty bias in response to sexual coercion. *Sex Roles, 31,* 387–405.

Struckman-Johnson, C., & Struckman-Johnson, D. (1997). Men's reactions to hypothetical forceful advances from women: The role of sexual standards, relationship availability, and the beauty bias. *Sex Roles, 37,* 319–333.

Struckman-Johnson, D., & Struckman-Johnson, C. (1996). College men's reactions to hypothetical forceful sexual advances from women. *Journal of Psychology and Human Sexuality, 8,* 93–105.

# 8

# Similar But Different: Men's and Women's Experiences of Sexual Coercion

E. SANDRA BYERS
LUCIA F. O'SULLIVAN

The words "sexual assault," "sexual aggression," and "sexual coercion" tend to conjure up an image of a male perpetrator and a female victim (Byers & O'Sullivan, 1996). In fact, for many people the concept of women's coercion of men seems ludicrous or, at most, extremely unlikely. There are a number of forces that maintain this stereotyped image. Most notable are factors related to gender role expectations. In particular, men's but not women's initiation of sexual activity and use of coercion is consistent with the traditional sexual script that prescribes appropriate gender roles for men and women in sexual situations. In keeping with perceptions of women's limited power in their interactions with men, there has been extensive research attention given to women's experiences of sexual

The contribution of the two authors is equal. Authorship order was determined alphabetically.

coercion and a corresponding neglect of research in which women are the initiators of sexual coercion. Researchers have clearly demonstrated that sexual coercion by a man is a common and serious problem for women that most often occurs within dating and other social relationships (Craig, 1990).[1]

Do men, in fact, always initiate sexual activity? Or do women sometimes take the more active and ardent role in sexual encounters? Is sexual coercion a problem that only women experience? Or is it also a problem for men? How are sexual coercion by men and by women similar? How are they different? Because the meaning of sexual coercion as experienced and perpetrated by men and women cannot be understood fully without examining the contexts in which coercion occurs, we begin with a discussion of beliefs associated with the typical sexually coercive event.

## SEXUAL COERCION AND THE TRADITIONAL SEXUAL SCRIPT

Several theorists have hypothesized that sexual coercion is caused by socialization practices that support antagonistic gender roles within the traditional sexual script and corresponding attitudes (Brownmiller, 1975; Clark & Lewis, 1977). According to the traditional sexual script, men are more highly motivated to engage in sexual activity than are women and pursue all opportunities to do so. On the other hand, women are expected to be sexually reluctant and responsible for setting firm limits in sexual encounters. Women are typically perceived as exchanging sex for attention or commitment rather than pursuing sex for its own sake. In contrast, sexual experience is seen as an important end in itself for men. Men's worth is enhanced by sexual experience; sexually experienced women are devalued. The traditional sexual script supports men's use of coercion if necessary to "convince" reluctant women to engage in sexual activity. Further, aggressiveness, instrumentality, and primary con-

[1] Although there is evidence that the incidence of sexual coercion among gay men and lesbian women is similar to that of heterosexual men and women (Waterman, Dawson, & Bologna, 1989), the following discussion is limited to heterosexual dating relationships. The research on same-sex relationships is too limited at this time to draw any definitive conclusions.

cern for one's own needs are part of traditional expectations for men but not for women. In short, the traditional sexual script in its most exaggerated form pits the oversexed, aggressive, emotionally insensitive male initiator who is enhanced by each sexual conquest and taught not to accept no for an answer against the unassertive, passive woman who is trying to protect her worth by restricting access to her sexuality while still appearing interested, sexy, and concerned about the man's needs (Byers, 1996).

The traditional sexual script is heterosexual and gender-schematized. That is, specific roles are assigned to men and others are assigned to women. Thus, it excludes the image of women as sexual aggressors, initiating sex with men, indicating their sexual interest, and, at times, coercing their reluctant partners to engage in unwanted sexual activities. Women are expected to influence men to avoid sex, not to have sex (Clark & Hatfield, 1989; McCormick, 1979). This script also excludes the image of men as sexually reluctant or as victims of sexual coercion. In fact, negative characteristics are ascribed to women and men who do not conform to the script: women who do not set limits within sexual relationships and men who do not push these limits. Media reports of sexual coercion most often conform to the stereotype of women as victims and men as aggressors. This is only in part because complaints to the police of sexual coercion are made almost exclusively by women. It also reflects widespread beliefs that sexual coercion of men by women is uncommon or impossible.

A number of researchers have examined beliefs about men's and women's differing sexual motives directly. Generally, they have done this by having participants rate, on a number of dimensions, vignettes describing coercive dating experiences with either a man or a woman as the victim. For example, participants might be asked to indicate how responsible the victim and/or perpetrator was for the assault or how pleasant the experience was for each. These studies indicate that gender stereotypes consistent with the traditional sexual script are prevalent among college students. For example, Smith, Pine, and Hawley (1988) found that male victims of sexual assault by a woman were rated as more likely to have encouraged the perpetrator and were viewed as experiencing less stress as a result of the experience than were female victims of male assault or same-gender assault victims. Male victims of women also were seen as experiencing the most pleasure from the assault.

Similarly, Garcia, Milano, and Quijano (1989) found that male victims of female coercion were judged to be more flattered and aroused, as well as less helpless and disgusted, by the coercive experience than were female victims of male coercion. That is, sexual coercion of men by women is generally viewed as less serious than sexual coercion of women by men. People tend to dismiss men's forced heterosexual sexual experiences as trivial or enjoyable, perhaps because they are so discordant with the stereotypic expectations delineated by the traditional sexual script.

Researchers also have been affected by the stereotypic expectations within the traditional sexual script. Although men's and women's behavior in sexual dating situations does not always conform to the traditional sexual script (e.g., Byers, 1996; O'Sullivan & Byers, 1992; Perper & Weis, 1987), most researchers examining sexual coercion have studied only women as victims and men as perpetrators. Typically, researchers have recruited both men and women as participants but simply asked both about their experiences or involvement in the sexual coercion of women by men (e.g., Koss & Oros, 1982; Koss, Gidycz, & Wisniewski, 1987). Until recently, women have rarely been asked about their use of coercion; men have rarely been asked about their experience of coercion. Limiting our investigations to this sexually coercive scenario perpetuates a restricted vision of the potential range of experiences that men and women might encounter.

Researchers have begun to examine where men and women cross the boundaries of expected behavior in sexually coercive dating encounters, thus removing the confound of victim–exploiter roles from gender (Lewin, 1985). In an early study, Sarrel and Masters (1982) described the experiences of several men seen in therapy, four of whom had been sexually coerced as adults by women. They found that not only did these men respond sexually under force (as some women do in coercive interactions) but also that there was a range of traumatic consequences associated with these coercive experiences. Other early investigations of men's and women's forced sexual experiences have confirmed that, in heterosexual relationships, men are sometimes victims of sexual coercion and women are sometimes perpetrators of sexual coercion (see Table 8.1). Further, these are not rare or isolated events, nor are they restricted to men seen in therapy. These results stand in stark contrast to the belief that, in heterosexual situations at least, men are the sole perpetrators of sexual coercion. Thus, the dynamics of sexually coercive interactions are more complex than researchers first realized.

In this chapter, we consider several important questions associated with comparisons of male and female experiences of sexual coercion. Before we address these questions, we examine some methodological issues related to estimating the prevalence of sexual coercion. Next, we review the prevalence of male and female sexual coercion in heterosexual relationships, as well as the prevalence of various types of sexual coercion. Then we examine similarities and differences in the circumstances of sexual coercion as perpetrated by men and by women. Finally, we compare the aftermath of coercive sexual experiences in terms of their psychosocial impact on victims of each gender.

## METHODOLOGICAL ISSUES IN DETERMINING THE PREVALENCE OF SEXUAL COERCION

Estimates of the prevalence of sexual coercion have varied considerably between studies (see Table 8.1). Between 22% and 83% of women report having been sexually coerced by a man (see Craig, 1990, for a review of prevalence studies), and between 4% and 44% of men report having experienced sexual coercion by a woman. Moreover, a smaller, but substantial, percentage of men (between 7% and 56%) and women (between 2% and 14%) acknowledge having engaged in sexual activity by using sexual coercion (Burke, Stets & Pirog-Good, 1988; Lane & Gwartney-Gibbs, 1985; or see Craig, 1990, for a review). How can we account for the wide variability in prevalence rates? What explanations might account for the discrepancies between prevalence rates based on victim reports and those based on perpetrator reports? These questions appear to be at the heart of many recent highly charged debates about the extent of sexual coercion in North American society.

### Variability in Estimates of the Prevalence of Sexual Coercion

Methodological differences between the studies may account for the wide variability in estimates of the prevalence of sexual coercion. Of particular importance is that researchers have differed in their operational definitions of sexual coercion. Specifically, the types of sexual activities assessed (e.g., intercourse only or the full range of sexual activities), the length of time assessed (e.g., lifetime experiences, experiences since age 14, experiences in the last year), and the sampling procedures used vary drastically across studies, making comparisons difficult (see Table 8.1).

Care needs to be taken when evaluating these findings. For example, use of the words "unwanted" or "unwilling" may be problematic in assessing sexual coercion, as these terms are not synonymous with "nonconsensual" or "forced" sexual activity. In contrast, the use of the terms "rape" or "acquaintance rape" may result in underreporting of sexual coercion because some respondents do not identify their nonconsensual experiences in these terms, particularly if the perpetrator was a trusted dating partner (Aizenman & Kelley, 1988; Baier, Rosenzweig, & Whipple, 1991; Koss & Oros, 1982). The variability in estimates of sexual coercion may also be attributed to researchers' use of instruments with unknown psychometric properties, so that the meaning of items is not known. Even the Sexual Experiences Survey, probably the mostly widely and most psychometrically sound instrument to measure sexual coercion, has been validated for men's use of coercion but not for women's use of coercion (Koss & Oros, 1982; Koss et al., 1987).

## Differences between Victimization and Perpetration Rates

Researchers have consistently noted that women's self-reports of sexual victimization by men are substantially higher than are men's self-reports of having victimized women. This discrepancy warrants concern because it calls into question the validity of self-reported coercion experiences. Moreover, this discrepancy has sometimes been interpreted as reflecting characteristics that are particular to men or to male socialization—a lack of awareness of their partner's reaction or reluctance to acknowledge coercive behavior. However, research on female coercion of men has found a parallel gender difference in prevalence rates, thus countering the argument that men alone are insensitive to their partner's wishes to refrain from sexual participation (Anderson & Aymami, 1993; O'Sullivan & Byers, 1993).

TABLE 8.1. Research Comparing Men's and Women's Participation in Coercive or Unwanted Sexual Activity

| | | | % Reporting | |
|---|---|---|---|---|
| Authors | Sample | Researchers' definition of coercive event | Men | Women |
| Aizenman & Kelley (1988) | 140 men 204 women Randomly selected undergraduate students | Involved in a situation they would call acquaintance rape | 6.0% | 22.0% |
| | | Successfully avoided such a situation | 18.0 | 51.0 |
| | | Forced to have intercourse against their will | 14.0 | 29.0 |
| | | Pressed to have unwanted sexual contact | 17.0 | 43.0 |
| Anderson & Aymami (1993) | 128 men 212 women Students from human sexuality classes at three institutions | For men: How many times has a woman attempted to have sexual contact with you by (recoded as none/1+) . . . For women: How many times have you attempted to have sexual contact with a man by (recoded as none/1+) . . . | 44.9% | 14.7% |
| | | Getting him drunk or stoned | 20.3 | 1.4 |
| | | Threatening self-harm | 29.9 | 11.3 |
| | | Pressuring with arguments | 15.6 | 3.8 |
| | | Threatening physical force | 15.6 | 5.7 |
| | | Using physical force | 18.0 | 8.5 |
| | | Threatening to end your relationship | 4.7 | 0.9 |
| | | Threatening with a weapon | | |
| Baier, Rosenzweig, & Whipple (1991) | 340 men 362 women Randomly selected college students | Misinterpreted level of sexual intimacy you desired | 51.9% | 73.4% |
| | | Person became so sexually aroused you felt it useless to stop him/her | 22.0 | 31.6 |
| | | Intercourse because he/she threatened to end relationship otherwise | 4.4 | 5.8 |
| | | Intercourse because felt pressured by continual arguments | 8.5 | 21.1 |
| | | Intercourse by saying things he/she didn't really mean | 14.9 | 24.9 |
| | | Physical force to try to make you engage in kissing or petting | 5.0 | 34.6 |
| | | Attempted intercourse by threatening to to use physical force | 0.9 | 11.9 |
| | | Attempted intercourse by using physical force | 1.8 | 18.8 |
| | | Intercourse because he/she threatened to use physical force | 0.9 | 5.8 |
| | | Intercourse because he/she used physical force | 1.2 | 11.9 |
| | | Sexual acts because threatened or used physical force | 0.6 | 4.1 |
| | | Have you ever been raped? | 0.9 | 7.2 |

| Study | Sample | Item | | (Means) |
|---|---|---|---|---|
| Burke, Stets, & Pirog-Good (1988) | 207 men 298 women Randomly selected upper-level college courses | Frequency with which you inflicted/ sustained a range of activities against your partner's/your will in the past year | | |
| | | Sustained minor sexual abuse (breast and genital fondling) | 0.8 | 1.8 |
| | | Sustained severe sexual abuse (attempted intercourse and intercourse) | 0.9 | 2.1 |
| | | Sustained sexual abuse (all forms) | 1.5 | 4.0 |
| | | Inflicted minor sexual abuse (breast and genital fondling) | 5.1 | 1.7 |
| | | Inflicted severe sexual abuse (attempted intercourse and intercourse) | 2.5 | 1.2 |
| | | Inflicted sexual abuse (all forms) | 7.0 | 2.6 |
| Erickson & Rapkin (1991) | 543 men 627 women Middle and high school students | Did you ever have a sexual experience (or sexual intercourse) with someone when you did not want to? | 12.0% | 18.0% |
| Hogben, Byrne, & Hamburger (1996) | 101 men 113 women College students | | | (Means) |
| | | Frequency with which you attempted to engage in [eight specific sexual behaviors] when your partner was not willing | 13.6 | 2.3 |
| | | Frequency with which a partner attempted to engage in [eight specific sexual behaviors] with you when you were not willing | 7.0 | 21.2 |
| | | Percentage reporting using one or more coercive behavior(s) | 41.0% | 24.0% |
| | | Percentage reporting one or more coercive experience(s) | 52.0 | 79.0 |
| Lane & Gwartney-Gibbs(1985) | 165 men 160 women Randomly selected college students | Have you ever been in a situation where . . . . | | |
| | | Intercourse because partner threatened to end relationship otherwise | 0.0% | 4.1% |
| | | Intercourse because felt pressured by continual arguments | 8.0 | 24.8 |
| | | Intercourse by saying things he/she didn't really mean | 5.1 | 17.0 |
| | | Intercourse unknowingly because you were very drunk, very "stoned" (on drugs), or unconscious | 12.8 | 12.5 |
| | | Threatened physical force to get you to engage in kissing, fondling, or intercourse | 1.1 | 5.3 |
| | | Used physical force to get you to engage in kissing, fondling, or intercourse | 1.6 | 12.9 |
| | | Used knife or gun to make you engage in kissing, fondling, or intercourse | 1.1 | 1.8 |
| | | You were raped | 1.1 | 4.6 |

(continued)

151

TABLE 8.1. (continued)

| Authors | Sample | Researchers' definition of coercive event | % Reporting | |
|---|---|---|---|---|
| | | | Men | Women |
| | | Intercourse because you threatened to end relationship otherwise | 3.9 | 0.9 |
| | | Intercourse because you continually pressured another with verbal arguments | 12.6 | 2.2 |
| | | Intercourse because you said things you didn't mean | 21.9 | 2.5 |
| | | Intercourse because you got a person very drunk, "stoned" (on drugs), or unconscious | 6.5 | 1.8 |
| | | Threatened to use physical force to make someone engage in kissing, fondling, or intercourse | 0.0 | 0.4 |
| | | Used physical force to make someone engage in kissing, fondling, or intercourse | 0.9 | 0.4 |
| | | Used a knife or gun to make someone engage in kissing, fondling, or intercourse | 0.0 | 0.0 |
| | | You raped someone | 0.0 | 0.0 |
| Lott, Reilly, & Howard (1982) | 377 men 542 women Randomly selected college students, staff, and faculty | Sexual contact through the use of force, threatened force, or a weapon, without consent, as inferred from refusal, helplessness, or incapacitation | 3.0% | 41.0% |
| | | Forced touching of intimate body parts | | |
| | | Penetration (vaginal, anal, or oral) | 0.0 | 11.0 |
| Muehlenhard & Cook (1988) | 507 men 486 women Introductory psychology students | Ever engaged in sexual activities (ranging from kissing to sexual intercourse) when you didn't really want to, either with or without pressure from the other person | | |
| | | Unwanted kissing, petting, or intercourse | 93.5% | 97.5% |
| | | Unwanted petting or intercourse | 83.8 | 84.0 |
| | | Unwanted intercourse | 62.7 | 46.3 |
| Poppen & Segal (1988) | 77 men 100 women Residence hall college students | Direct actions to induce one's partner to engage in a behavior that he/she might otherwise resist | | |
| | | Initiated passionate kissing | 30.0% | 12.0% |
| | | Initiated genital touching | 30.0 | 2.0 |
| | | Initiated oral sex | 30.0 | 2.0 |
| | | Initiated sexual intercourse | 38.0 | 1.0 |

| Study | Sample | Question/Behavior | Men | Women |
|---|---|---|---|---|
| | | Initiated any of these behaviors | 56.0 | 14.0 |
| | | Experienced passionate kissing | 36.0 | 51.0 |
| | | Experienced genital touching | 14.0 | 38.0 |
| | | Experienced oral sex | 12.0 | 40.0 |
| | | Experienced sexual intercourse | 18.0 | 37.0 |
| | | Experienced any of these behaviors | 44.0 | 74.0 |
| Sandberg, Jackson, & Petretic-Jackson (1987) | 161 men 247 women Introductory psychology students | Have you ever felt a dating partner provoked sexually aggressive behavior in you by refusing reasonable sexual requests? | 65.0% | 61.0% |
| | | Have you ever felt verbally pressured by a dating partner to have sexual intercourse? | 48.0 | 74.0 |
| | | Have you ever been sexually assaulted by a dating partner consisting of being touched, held, or kissed against your will? | 25.0 | 48.0 |
| | | Have you ever been physically forced by a dating partner to have sexual intercourse? | 6.0 | 21.0 |
| | | Have you ever been sexually abused in any way in a dating relationship? | 0.0 | 8.0 |
| | | Have you ever been sexually abusive to your dating partner in a dating relationship? | 2.0 | 1.0 |
| Sorenson & Siegel (1992) | More than 1,410 men More than 1,590 women Randomly selected L.A. community residents | In your lifetime, has anyone ever tried to pressure or force you to have sexual contact? By sexual contact, I mean their touching of your sexual parts, your touching their sexual parts, or sexual intercourse? | 9.4% | 16.7% |
| Struckman-Johnson (1988) | 268 men 355 women Psychology and residence hall college students | In the course of your life, how many times have you been forced to engage in sexual intercourse while on a date? Give a number from 0 – . | 16.0% | 22.0% |
| | | In the course of your life, how many times have you forced someone to engage in sexual intercourse while on a date? Give a number from 0 – . | 10.0 | 2.0 |

153

Within a broader framework, O'Sullivan and Byers (1996) found that both men and women attributed the use of more negative (including coercive) strategies to influence a reluctant partner to engage in sexual activity to the other gender than they attributed to themselves.

There are several possible reasons for the discrepancy between reports of using and experiencing sexually coercive behaviors. None of these studies used dating couples as participants. Thus, the men and the women in the studies were not partners and may come from separate dating populations that differ in the prevalence of sexual coercion. If so, the prevalence estimates, although different, may both be accurate. It is also possible that these discrepancies reflect a self-enhancing or self-protective tendency to overlook or disregard our most reprehensible behavior. Alternately, they may reflect an actor–observer bias—the reluctant partner has access to his or her own thoughts and feelings, to which the ardent partner does not have access. Similarly, the ardent partner has access to his or her "true" intentions, whereas the reluctant partner would be relying solely on his or her own judgments of the partner's overt behavior. This may lead to differences in perceptions of what occurred during the sexual encounter.

## Meaning of Prevalence Data

Most of the research has assessed the *prevalence* of sexual coercion (the proportion of the population that has ever experienced coercion) rather than the incidence of sexual coercion (how many individuals experience sexual coercion within a specific period of time). Some theorists have concluded, incorrectly, from prevalence data that most dating interactions are sexually coercive, whereas this is actually a statement about the incidence of sexual coercion (e.g., Clark & Lewis, 1977; Roiphe, 1993). To what extent is sexual coercion typical or normative of dating interactions? Is sexual coercion commonly used to resolve sexual disagreements?

Although many women have been sexually coerced at some point in the past, only a small minority of dates involve sexual coercion (Byers & Lewis, 1988). In fact, by far the most likely outcome in situations in which there is a discrepancy in the desired level of sexual activity is that the more ardent partner complies without question with his or her partner's reluctance to engage in the sexual activity (Byers, 1988; Byers & Lewis, 1988; Byers & Wilson, 1985; O'Sullivan & Byers, 1993, 1996). This is true of both men and women. Moreover, in situations in which men or women do try to influence their partners to engage in unwanted sexual activity, most of their influence strategies are experienced as positive and noncoercive rather than as negative and coercive (O'Sullivan & Byers, 1993, 1996). Although a substantial percentage of women and men have experienced sexual coercion, use of sexual coercion in dating situations is not typical for either women or men (Byers, 1996).

In sum, interpretation of research on the prevalence of male and female sexual coercion is hampered by several methodological short-comings, as well as by a lack of a consistent methodology. Awareness of methodological issues may prevent misinterpretation of the data and promote greater scientific rigor—so crucial in this highly politicized field. In particular, we need to ensure that findings based on the prevalence of sexual coercion are not used to draw erroneous conclusions about sexual interactions in general.

## COMPARISON OF THE PREVALENCE OF MALE AND FEMALE SEXUAL COERCION

Despite methodological variation, the results of research comparing the prevalence of male and female sexual coercion are surprisingly consistent. In keeping with the traditional sexual script, researchers almost uniformly have found that more women than men report having experienced sexual coercion and more men than women report having used sexual coercion. (See Table 8.1 for a summary of studies examining prevalence rates.) For example, with Larry Finkelman, we surveyed 1,454 randomly selected undergraduate students at two Canadian universities about their sexual coercion experiences during the previous academic year (Byers, O'Sullivan, & Finkelman, 1996; O'Sullivan, Byers, & Finkelman, 1998). Usable questionnaires were received from 434 (29.8%) students, of which data from 216 unmarried women and 130 unmarried men were analyzed further. The questionnaire was designed to assess the types, frequency, charac-teristics, and aftermath of coercive sexual experiences that had occurred during the previous academic year. The frequency of use and experience of sexual coercion was assessed on separate sections of the questionnaire using the operational definitions provided by Koss et al. (1987) in the Sexual Experiences Survey, reworded to be gender-neutral. Respondents who reported one or more coercive sexual experiences also responded to a series of questions about the coercive sexual incident in which they had experienced the highest level of pressure or force. Consistent with past research, we found that more women (42.5%) than men (18.5%) reported one or more coercive sexual experiences (O'Sullivan et al., 1998). Similarly, more men (20.0%) than women (8.8%) reported using some form of sexual coercion. In one of the few studies that did not use college students, Sorenson and Siegel (1992) found that significantly more women than men residing in Los Angeles reported that someone had pressured or forced them to have sexual contact at some point in their lives. This was true regardless of the ethnicity, age, or educational level of the respondent.

In sum, these studies indicate that women do use sexual coercion in their relationships with men. A substantial proportion of men report having engaged in unwanted sexual activity as a result of women's use of coercion, and a smaller, but still notable, percentage of women report having used coercion. Nonetheless, sexual coercion appears to be a more prevalent problem for women than it is for men.

## TYPES OF SEXUAL COERCION

Several researchers have investigated whether the gender difference in rates of experience and use of sexual coercion is true of all types of coercive sexual experiences. Most researchers have found that more women than men report each of a wide range of coercive experiences. Further, men do not report experiencing any coercive behaviors more frequently than do women (Baier et al., 1991; Muehlenhard & Cook, 1988; Poppen & Segal, 1988). For example, we found that women reported having experienced each of the ten coercive sexual experiences listed on the Sexual Experiences Survey more frequently than did men, including both unwanted sex play and intercourse as a result of physical coercion, threat of force, and force (O'Sullivan et al., in press). Reports of unwanted sexual activity as a result of being given alcohol or drugs did not differ statistically, however. Similarly, Poppen and Segal (1988) found that more women than men reported having experienced four of five coercive sexual strategies to initiate sex. Further, they found that more men than women reported having used each of the coercive strategies and behaviors.

Some researchers have asked participants to describe their most recent forced-sex episode as a way of comparing the types of coercion typically experienced by men and women. The incidents described by women are more likely than those described by men to involve physical harm. For example, Struckman-Johnson (1988) found that the type of sexual coercion most frequently reported by female victims was physical force (55% of women vs. 10% of males), whereas the type of coercion most frequently reported by men was psychological pressure (16% of women compared to 52% of men). Sorenson and Siegel (1992) found that, compared to men, women who had experienced sexual coercion were more likely to be harmed or threatened with harm. In contrast, men who had experienced sexual coercion were more likely to have been verbally pressured for sexual contact.

In sum, the finding that more women than men experience sexual coercion and more men than women use sexual coercion is not confined to one or a few coercive experiences but is consistent across a wide range of sexual experiences and coercive strategies. Further, more women than men experience severe forms of sexual coercion. Thus, to answer one of the most important questions addressed in this chapter: Sexual coercion is not a problem for women only, as some men also experience sexual coercion in their dating relationships. However, sexual coercion is more of a problem for women than for men, using the probability of experiencing sexual coercion and the severity of these coercive acts to evaluate the extent of the problem.

## CIRCUMSTANCES ASSOCIATED WITH MEN'S AND WOMEN'S EXPERIENCES OF SEXUAL COERCION

The typical incident of a man's sexual coercion of a woman occurs in the context of an ongoing relationship; often the victim is romantically interested in the perpetrator (Aizenman & Kelley, 1988; Miller & Marshall, 1987). Are the circumstances the same when women sexually coerce a male partner? Or does the context of male and female sexual coercion differ in some important ways?

There is little research addressing the context in which sexual coercion of men by women occurs. However, in our study of male and female sexual coercion, we examined the circumstances surrounding sexually coercive experiences (O'Sullivan et al., 1998). We had victims of sexual coercion provide information about the characteristics and context of the sexually coercive situation that involved the most extreme level of pressure or force that they had experienced in the preceding year. For the most part, the women's and the men's descriptions of the sexually coercive situations did not differ. Typically, the sexual coercion was committed by a person known to the victim—either a current dating partner (44.2%) or acquaintance (36.5%). In keeping with the typical heterosexual dating script (Rose & Frieze, 1993), we found that, reportedly, most offenders and victims had been using drugs or alcohol, most acts of sexual coercion occurred late in the evening in either the victim's or the perpetrator's room or apartment (more often in the woman's), and most victims had engaged in some type of consensual sex with the perpetrator on a previous occasion or on the day of the unwanted incident. The most frequently reported nonconsensual sexual activity was intercourse, followed by kissing. More than a third of both the men and the women reported that this was not the first time the perpetrator had used sexual coercion. Our findings are consistent with both a large body of research examining the context of men's sexual coercion of women and the few studies examining women's sexual coercion of men. That is, the sexual coercion of both young, single men and young, single women typically occurs within the dating context (Aizenman & Kelley, 1988; Byers & Eastman, 1979; Kanin, 1985; Lott, Reilly, & Howard, 1982; Miller & Marshall, 1987; Muehlenhard & Linton, 1987; O'Sullivan & Byers, 1996).

The two most frequently coercive strategies reported by both the men and the women were use of continual arguments and pleading, and ignoring requests to stop. Compared to the women, the men more often reported having been drugged or given too much to drink. The men and women did not differ in the frequency with which they reported 13 other strategies, ranging from less coercive means (e.g., continual arguments and pleading) to more coercive means (e.g., injury from a weapon).

In sum, the circumstances and contexts of sexual coercion of men and women are, for the most part, extremely similar. Sexual coercion, both by women and by men, appears to occur typically in the context of a dating relationship. As such, sexual coercion often occurs after some level of consensual sexual activity and in a private setting. Sexual intercourse is the most frequently experienced non-consensual sexual activity, often accompanied by unwanted kissing. Use of coercion is frequently, although not typically, a pattern in these relationships, as a substantial minority of respondents reported that this was not the first time their partners had used sexual coercion. Although there were a few differences in the frequency with which the various coercive strategies were used, for the most part it appears that women adopt the same strategies to coerce a reluctant partner that men do. Similarly, Byers (1996) concluded, more generally, that men's and women's roles in sexual interactions overlap considerably, particularly in established relationships.

## AFTERMATH OF MALE AND FEMALE SEXUAL COERCION

As we have seen, both men and women experience sexual coercion in their dating relationships, and, superficially at least, these experiences appear similar. However, this does not mean that men's and women's experiences of sexual coercion are the same. To understand the meaning of sexually coercive experiences, it is necessary to take a phenomenological perspective. That is, we cannot assume a priori the (negative) consequences of nonconsensual sexual activity. Rather, we need to have men and women describe the aftermath of their experiences for themselves. This is especially important in light of the fact that many respondents do not label their nonconsensual sexual experiences as "sexual coercion" or "sexual assault." The labeling of these events as sexual coercion is researcher-imposed. Therefore, a final, and perhaps the most important, question in comparing male and female coercive sexual experiences is whether the impact of sexual coercion in heterosexual adult relationships is comparable for men and women. That is, even though the activities, circumstances, and contexts of the nonconsensual experiences appear to be similar for men and women, the meaning given to and the psychological response to coercive sex may differ in crucial ways. Outside of this phenomenological context, statistics about the rates and types of sexually coercive experiences are not a meaningful way of defining this social problem.

## Responses to Sexual Coercion

Few researchers have examined the impact of sexual coercion in nonclinical samples, particularly for men. Most women have a strong negative reaction to coercive sexual experiences (Byers & Eastman, 1979; Calhoun, Atkeson, & Resick, 1982; Koss, Dinero, Seibel, & Cox, 1988). Sarrel and Masters' (1982) case studies demonstrate that men, too, can be traumatized by sexually coercive experiences. However, as might be expected, men tend to rate their likely reactions to unwanted sexual advances by a woman as less negative (and barely negative) than women rate their (very negative) reactions to unwanted sexual advances by a man when judging hypothetical situations (Struckman-Johnson, 1988; Struckman-Johnson & Struckman-Johnson, 1993). This is particularly true if the advances are made by a dating partner (Struckman-Johnson & Struckman-Johnson, 1996). In fact, some men believed that their reactions to the unexpected sexual advance by a woman would be positive. Presumably, these latter incidents were interpreted by men as a noncoercive expression of sexual desire, even though they involved unexpected, forceful sexual touching.

Assessing beliefs about how men and women think they will react in a coercive situation may tell us more about their endorsement of stereotypes about sexual coercion than about how they would actually react in that situation. To bypass this problem, we examined several reactions to experiences of sexual coercion by men and women, including their behavioral responses to their partners, their emotional reactions to the event, its impact on other aspects of their lives, and their reporting of the event (O'Sullivan et al., 1998). Both the men and the women reported resisting the perpetrator's attempts to gain compliance, being clear in their communication of their unwillingness to engage in the sexual activity, and believing that the perpetrator understood that they were unwilling to engage in the sexual activity. Thus, unlike hypothetical scenarios, their reactions suggest that the situations described by both the men and the women were nonconsensual rather than merely unexpected. Nonetheless, compared to the men, the women were more likely to report responses indicative of a strong adverse reaction to the unwanted advances.

Compared to the men, the women reported being more upset by the incident, both at the time it occurred and at the time of the survey. For example, 31.3% of the women but only 14.3% of the men reported being extremely upset by the coercive experience. More women than men indicated that they used strong resistance strategies, such as becoming hostile and angry, screaming, yelling, and/or physically resisting and fighting back, in response to their partner's coercive behavior. In addition, compared to the men, the women rated themselves as more clearly indicating to their partner their unwillingness to engage in the sexual activity. The women more often reported believing that the perpetrator understood their unwillingness to engage in the sexual activity.

These results suggest that women see the possibility of engaging in unwanted sexual activity as more adverse than do men and are more likely to view their partner's behavior as knowingly coercive. Moreover, women react more strongly than do men when faced with a partner who is attempting to pressure or force them to engage in an unwanted sexual activity. Similarly, in their community sample, Sorenson and Siegel (1992) found that although anger was the most common emotional reaction of both men and women, a significantly greater proportion of women than men reported experiencing 11 of the 15 negative emotional and behavioral responses to sexual assault. These emotions included fear, stopping previous activities, fear of sex, loss of sexual interest, decrease in sexual pleasure, feeling dishonored or spoiled, sadness or depression, anger, tension or anxiety, insomnia, and fear of being alone. In addition, women were more likely than were men to use physical resistance strategies.

However, in our study, not all respondents reported adverse reactions to the coercive sexual experience (O'Sullivan et al., 1998). For example, 42.9% of the men and 6.3% of the women reported being not at all upset by the incident at the time it occurred. Most research, including our own, has used instruments that operationally define the experiences but do not require respondents to label them as sexual coercion or sexual assault. Thus, it is unclear whether the respondents who report not being distressed by the experience are, in fact, "hidden victims" who have not yet recognized and labeled their own victimization. Alternately, perhaps we need to be careful about a priori interpretation of these experiences as coercive experiences for the victim. In fact, O'Sullivan and Byers (1993) found that none of the behaviors used to try to influence a reluctant partner to engage in sexual activity were considered negative by all respondents who had experienced them, including such strategies as ignoring the refusal, sulking, and pleading. Influence strategies that were rated as having a negative impact by some respondents were rated as having a neutral or positive impact by other respondents. Thus, the same behavior may have a different impact on different people.

## Life Changes Following Sexual Coercion

In addition to investigating respondents' immediate emotional and behavioral reactions to the sexually coercive experience, we also investigated the impact of the sexual coercion on their lives (O'Sullivan et al., 1998). About one-fifth of the men and the women reported that the incident decreased their involvement in job, community, sports, or social activities, whereas approximately one-third indicated that the incident decreased their ability to concentrate, complete course assignments, take exams, or attend lectures. About half of the men and the women reported that they had told someone about the incident, most often a friend. Few men or women had reported it to a person in authority. Sorenson and Siegel (1992) also found no difference in men's and women's likelihood to report the event, although they did find that women were more likely than were men to talk to a mental health professional, a physician, or the police.

In sum, these results suggest that women are generally more distressed by coercive sexual experiences than are men. The similarity in men's and women's reports of the characteristics and circumstances of sexual coercion does not imply that these experiences have the same meaning and impact on men and women. In general, sexual coercion appears to be a more adverse experience for women than it is for men. Nonetheless, for some men, being coerced to engage in some type of sexual activity is extremely upsetting. Thus, we should not ignore nor trivialize the reality of these men's experiences of sexual coercion by women.

## CONCLUSIONS

At the beginning of this chapter we posed the question about the extent to which men's and women's experiences of sexual coercion are similar or different. Formulations of sexual coercion based on traditional sexual scripts predict sharp distinctions between men's and women's behavior in sexual situations. According to this traditional view, there is little or no expectation of women's abuse of power in sexual relationships. In essence, sexual coercion in dating relationships is seen to lie exclusively in the realm of women's experiences. It would rarely, if ever, be a problem for men. A review of the literature of men's and women's experiences of sexual coercion indicates the following:

1. Both women and men use sexual coercion. However, sexual coercion is a more prevalent experience for women than it is for men. Women are more likely to experience each of the full range of sexually coercive behaviors than are men.

2. For the most part, when sexual coercion does occur, the circumstances are similar for men and women. These circumstances are characteristic of the common dating script.

3. When women use coercion against men, they tend to adopt similar behaviors in similar situations as do men. The sharp distinctions between appropriate behavior for men and women in sexual dating situations based on the traditional sexual script are missing.

4. The aftermath of sexual coercion tends to differ for men and women. In general, as indicated by their reports of both their behavior and emotional reactions, women are more distressed after an experience of sexual coercion than are men. However, not all women (or men) report being upset by nonconsensual sexual experiences.

5. Some men report substantial distress in response to sexual coercion by a woman.

What are the implications of these findings for researchers, therapists, and educators? First, the finding that both men and women experience sexual coercion suggests that we need to expand our knowledge in this area. We should not let our assumptions based on gender-role stereotypes unduly influence the research questions we ask or our ability to prevent sexual coercion by either gender. We need to incorporate information about both genders into our designs of education, prevention, and treatment programs and to ensure that we do not unfairly stereotype one gender. It is important to restore balance in our understanding of sexual coercion and of gender. Women are not always victims; men are not always aggressors. Compared to some women, some men are as distressed or more distressed by their experiences. Some women and some men are not particularly distressed by nonconsensual sexual experiences.

Second, we need to reconsider some of our assumptions about the causes of sexual coercion. It may be that sexual coercion often is not a consequence of gender scripts. Rather, it is a consequence of a sexual script in which communication is poor and myths about sexual rights and proprieties abound. In the absence of effective communication, men's assumptions that women's indications of reluctance usually constitute token refusals may contribute to sexual coercion in that men will tend to disbelieve women's genuine refusals. Similarly, in the absence of effective communication, women's belief in the cultural myth that men are always interested in and ready to engage in sex and that it is therefore impossible to sexually victimize a male dating partner may also contribute to sexual coercion. We cannot neglect to educate both men and women about the need to recognize and respect their partner's wishes. We need to give men and women the skills and the comfort to communicate about their sexual relationship effectively.

Third, the finding that sexual coercion is more of a problem for women than for men in its frequency, severity, and impact means that we need to continue to consider sexual coercion by men and women separately in our research and in our prevention programs. For the most part, men's and women's experiences of sexual coercion are superficially similar but substantively different. As women in our society generally have less power in relationships with men and are physically weaker, women may be more inclined than are men to view a coercive attempt as threatening to their physical and emotional security.

Finally, a goal of sexual science should be to promote men's and women's recognition of events that do not allow their full expression of the right to choose sexual participation. A decision to engage in sex should be based on an assessment of self-enhancing benefits. Both men and women should have the freedom to decline unwanted sexual opportunities and know that their partner will respect their choice to do so. This can only be attained by challenging stereotypes, promoting knowledge and awareness, and improving communication skills.

## REFERENCES

Aizenman, M., & Kelley, G. (1988). The incidence of violence and acquaintance rape in dating relationships among college men and women. *Journal of College Student Development, 29,* 305–311.

Anderson, P. , & Aymami, R. (1993). Reports of female initiation of sexual contact: Male and female differences. *Archives of Sexual Behavior, 22,* 335–343.

Baier, J., Rosenzweig, M., & Whipple, E. (1991). Patterns of sexual behavior, coercion, and victimization of university students. *Journal of College Student Development, 32,* 310–322.

Brownmiller, S. (1975). *Against our will: Men, women, and rape.* New York: Simon & Schuster.

Burke, P., Stets, J., & Pirog-Good, M. (1988). Gender identity, self-esteem, and physical and sexual abuse in dating relationships. *Social Psychology Quarterly, 51,* 272–285.

Byers, E. (1988). Effects of sexual arousal on men and women's behavior in sexual disagreement situations. *Journal of Sex Research, 25,* 235–254.

Byers, E. (1996). How well does the traditional sexual script explain sexual coercion? Review of a program of research. *Journal of Psychology and Human Sexuality, 8,* 6–26.

Byers, E., & Eastman, M. (1979, June). *Characteristics of unreported sexual assaults.* Paper presented at the meeting of the Canadian Psychological Association, Quebec City, Quebec, Canada.

Byers, E., & Lewis, K. (1988). Dating couples' disagreements over the desired level of sexual activity. *Journal of Sex Research, 24,* 15–29.

Byers, E., & O'Sullivan, L. (1996). Introduction. *Journal of Psychology and Human Sexuality, 8,* 1–5.

Byers, E. S., O'Sullivan, L. F., & Finkelman, L. (1996, April). *Broadening sexual coercion research: Characteristics and impact of men's and women's use of sexual coercion.* Paper presented at the Western Region meeting of the Society for the Scientific Study of Sex, San Diego, CA.

Byers, E., & Wilson, P. (1985). Accuracy of women's expectations regarding men's responses to refusals of sexual advances in dating situations. *International Journal of Women's Studies, 4,* 376–387.

Calhoun, K., Atkeson, B. M., & Resick, P. A. (1982). A longitudinal examination of fear reactions in victims of rape. *Journal of Counseling Psychology, 29,* 655–661.

Clark, R., & Hatfield, E. (1989). Gender differences in receptivity to sexual offers. *Journal of Psychology and Human Sexuality, 2,* 39–55.

Clark, L., & Lewis, D. (1977). *Rape: The price of coercive sexuality.* Toronto, Ontario, Canada: The Woman's Press.

Craig, M. (1990). Coercive sexuality in dating relationships: A situational model. *Clinical Psychology Review, 10,* 395–423.

Erickson, P., & Rapkin, A. (1991). Unwanted sexual experiences among middle and high-school youth. *Journal of Adolescent Health, 12,* 319–325.

Garcia, L., Milano, L., & Quijano, A. (1989). Perceptions of coercive sexual behavior by males and females. *Sex Roles, 21,* 569–577.

Hogben, M., Byrne, D., & Hamburger, M. (1996). Coercive heterosexuality in dating relationships of college students: Implications of differential male–female experience. *Journal of Psychology and Human Sexuality, 8,* 69–78.

Kanin, E. (1985). Date rapists: Differential sexual socialization and relative deprivation. *Archives of Sexual Behavior, 14,* 219–231.

Koss, M., Dinero, T., Seibel, C., & Cox, S. (1988). Stranger and acquaintance rape: Are there differences in victim's experience? *Psychology of Women Quarterly, 12,* 1–24.

Koss, M., Gidycz, C., & Wisniewski, N. (1987). The scope of rape: Incidence and prevalence of sexual aggression and victimization in a national sample of higher education students. *Journal of Consulting and Clinical Psychology, 55,* 162–170.

Koss, M., & Oros, C. (1982). Sexual Experiences Survey: A research instrument investigating sexual aggression and victimization. *Journal of Consulting and Clinical Psychology, 50,* 455–457.

Lane, K., & Gwartney-Gibbs, P. (1985). Violence in the context of dating and sex. *Journal of Family Issues, 6,* 45–59.

Lewin, M. (1985). Unwanted intercourse: The difficulty of saying no. *Psychology of Women Quarterly, 9,* 184–192.

Lott, B., Reilly, M., & Howard, D. (1982). Sexual assault and harassment: A campus community case study. *Signs: Journal of Woman in Culture and Society, 8,* 296–319.

McCormick, N. (1979). Come-ons and put-offs: Unmarried students' strategies for having and avoiding sexual intercourse. *Psychology of Women Quarterly, 4,* 194–211.

Miller, B., & Marshall, J. (1987). Coercive sex on the university campus. *Journal of College Student Personnel, 28,* 38–47.

Muehlenhard, C., & Cook, S. (1988). Men's self-reports of unwanted sexual activity. *Journal of Sex Research, 24,* 58–72.

Muehlenhard, C., & Linton, M. (1987). Date rape and sexual aggression in dating situations: Incidence and risk factors. *Journal of Counseling Psychology, 34,* 186–196.

O'Sullivan, L., & Byers, E. (1992). College students' incorporation of initiator and restrictor roles in sexual dating interactions. *Journal of Sex Research, 29,* 435–446.

O'Sullivan, L., & Byers, E. (1993). Eroding stereotypes: College women's attempts to influence reluctant male sexual partners. *Journal of Sex Research, 30,* 270–282.

O'Sullivan, L., & Byers, E. (1996). Gender differences in responses to discrepancies in desired level of sexual intimacy. *Journal of Psychology and Human Sexuality, 8,* 49–67.

O'Sullivan, L., Byers, E., & Finkelman, L. (1998). A comparison of male and female college students' experiences of sexual coercion. *Psychology of Women Quarterly.*

Perper, T., & Weis, D. (1987). Proceptive and rejective strategies of U.S. and Canadian college women. *Journal of Sex Research, 23,* 455–480.

Poppen, P., & Segal, N. (1988). The influence of sex and sex role orientation on sexual coercion. *Sex Roles, 19,* 689–701.

Roiphe, K. (1993). *The morning after: Sex, fear, and feminism on campus.* Boston: Little, Brown.

Rose, S., & Frieze, I. (1993). Young singles' contemporary dating scripts. *Sex Roles, 28,* 499–509.

Sandberg, G., Jackson, T., & Petretic-Jackson, P. (1987). College students' attitudes regarding sexual coercion and aggression: Developing educational and preventive strategies. *Journal of College Student Personnel, 28,* 302–311.

Sarrel, P., & Masters, W. (1982). Sexual molestation of men by women. *Archives of Sexual Behavior, 11,* 117–131.

Smith, R., Pine, C., & Hawley, M. (1988). Social cognition about adult male victims of female sexual assault. *Journal of Sex Research, 24,* 101–112.

Sorenson, S., & Siegel, J. (1992). Gender, ethnicity, and sexual assault: Findings from a Los Angeles study. *Journal of Social Issues, 48,* 93–104.

Struckman-Johnson, C. (1988). Forced sex on dates: It happens to men, too. *Journal of Sex Research, 24,* 234–241.

Struckman-Johnson, C., & Struckman-Johnson, D. (1993). College men's and women's reactions to hypothetical sexual touch varied by initiator gender and coercion level. *Sex Roles, 29,* 373–387.

Struckman-Johnson, D., & Struckman-Johnson, C. (1996). College men's reactions to hypothetical forceful sexual advances from women. *Journal of Psychology and Human Sexuality, 8,* 93–105.

Waterman, C., Dawson, L., & Bologna, M. (1989). Sexual coercion in gay male and lesbian relationships: Predictors and implications for support services. *Journal of Sex Research, 26,* 118–124.

# 9

# Women's Sexual Coercion of Men: A Feminist Analysis

## WENDY STOCK

## MALE AND FEMALE EXPERIENCES OF FORCED SEX: SIMILARITIES AND DIFFERENCES

Debate in the area of female sexual aggression against men turns on the extent to which this phenomenon is comparable to male sexual aggression against women. Some feminists have contended that sexual aggression is not gender-neutral, stressing the importance of gender in social context and relative access to power. A behavioral description and review of the physical and psychological sequelae of these experiences is a first step toward resolving the question of equivalency of male-to-female and female-to-male sexual aggression. First, a brief overview of several representative studies illustrates the misapplication of research on male rape. The second half of this chapter contextualizes the misuse of research on male rape within the backlash against feminism.

As noted by Struckman-Johnson (1988), reports of sexual victimization against men have been on the increase since the 1970s. Most male victims treated at rape centers have usually been assaulted by other men. However, it has been contended that men may be reluctant to report sexual aggression by women (Sarrel & Masters, 1982) due to embarrassment and deviation from the perceived male gender role of sexual invulnerability and control. Although it is most probable that male sexual victimization by women is significantly underreported, a discussion of prevalence rates is beyond the scope of this chapter. What happens in a typical "male rape" by a woman? Struckman-Johnson (1988) surveyed male and female college students and compared descriptions of forced-sex episodes in dating situations. Among 268 men in her sample, 43 (16%) reported that they had been forced to engage in sexual intercourse on a date. Of the 355 women surveyed, 79 (22%) reported that they had been forced to engage in sexual intercourse on a date at least once during their lifetimes. A significant proportion of men (10%) stated that they had forced sex on a date at least once in their lifetimes, compared to 2% of the women.

Men and women reported significantly different experiences of the type of coercion used to obtain sex. Most men reported coercion into sex by psychological tactics, through verbal pressure by their partners, and in order to avoid guilt over disappointing their partners. In several cases the men were blackmailed by their girlfriends, who threatened to end their relationship unless sex was provided. Two others were blackmailed by threats of exposure of embarrassing information to others. Twenty-eight percent of the men were forced into sex by a combination of psychological and physical pressure. The men's accounts described women partners engaging in unwanted sexual touching ("coming on heavily") and refusing to stop when asked, with the men eventually giving in. In no cases did it appear, in accounts cited by Struckman-Johnson (1988), that a man was actually physically unable to escape.

In contrast to the men, most women (55%) reported being physically forced. Typical descriptions included physical force and inability to escape. Nineteen percent of the women were coerced by a combination of psychological tactics and physical restraint.

Emotional sequelae for men and women differed significantly, in terms of both immediate and long-term reactions. Most women's immediate and long-term reactions were negative, with the most common aftereffect being wariness around men. Forty-four percent of the men felt neutral immediately after the incident, with the remainder divided between feeling positive and negative.

Although Struckman-Johnson (1988) concludes that both men and women engage in sexually exploitative behaviors, ranging from verbal pressure to use of physical force and restraint, the proportions of men and women using these strategies varied significantly. The most typical experience reported by the vast majority of men was engaging in sex to avoid guilt and disappointment of their partners. These descriptions sound uncannily familiar, describing the "normal" conditions under which many women engage in sex in their heterosexual dating and marital relationships. In fact, Muehlenhard and Cook (1988) reported that significantly more women engaged in unwanted sexual activity for "altruistic" reasons, although both genders reported this reason at fairly high rates (87% women and 72% men). In the same study, significantly fewer men engaged in unwanted sexual activity because they felt obligated. Although engaging in unwanted sexual activity for any reason is not desirable, it is important to differentiate reasons such as feeling obligated, not wanting to reject a sexual partner, and altruism from forms of sexual coercion in which the individual has, physically, no choice.

The men in Struckman-Johnson's study reported no instances in which actual physical restraint was used by women against them. The most extreme examples provided included a few men who had unwanted sex while intoxicated: "She layed [*sic*] on top of me when I was drunk and took my clothing off and went to work" (1988, p. 239). However, it seems likely that this man could have managed to escape if the house was on fire, despite his inebriated state. Another wrote that a woman grabbed his penis and would not let go until he had sex. Anatomically speaking, his partner had to let go of his penis at some point in order to accomplish sexual intercourse, a criterion in this study. At this point he could have escaped. Another man had sex with a woman who was driving the car in order to avoid a potentially long walk home had he refused. In contrast, the women's accounts showed a predominance of physical force used, with physical restraint used against 19% of the women. In most situations in which physical force is reported, most men are significantly larger and stronger and are able to walk out if they choose, whereas physical resistance by women in the same situation is often ineffective and futile. This would suggest very different subjective experiences of unwanted sexual activity due to physical coercion in men and women.

Traumatic experiences tend to have severe and negative short-

and long-term impact. If male-to-female and female-to-male forced sex is equivalent, it would be expected that men and women would report equal degrees of negative emotional sequelae. Among the women, 78% reported negative long-term impact, compared to 22% of men. Perhaps if a greater proportion of the men had experienced physical force/restraint, these rates would be more similar. However, they did not. These data do not support Struck-man-Johnson's characterization of "the one-sided presentation of female forced sex incidence rates," which fosters perceptions of men as aggressive and women as passive victims. Instead, the data indicate that men do use higher levels of aggression to obtain sexual access to women. Women use less physically coercive influence strategies, from which escape by the putative victim is more often possible, with male victims suffering, in general, less psychological trauma.

Certainly, the traditional stereotype of women as nondesirous of sex is challenged by the range of some of the approaches described in Struckman-Johnson. Another study by O'Sullivan and Byers (1993) found that college students' experiences of situations that are characterized by a woman desiring a higher level of sexual activity than does her male partner is not uncommon among this popula-tion. A number of active initiating strategies were used by women with reluctant male partners, but predominantly participants indi-cated that the woman complied with the man's refusals and used no influence behaviors. However, even if women sometimes take the initiative sexually and use low levels of verbal coercion, this does not obviate the fact that men tend to use higher levels of aggression, nor does it remove the differences in concrete power (physical strength) that make the playing field of dating sex uneven.

Muehlenhard and Cook (1988) also investigated men's experi-ence of unwanted sexual activity, defined as unwanted kissing, petting, or intercourse. Interestingly, more men (62.7%) than women (46.3%) had experienced unwanted intercourse, although more women than men had experienced unwanted sexual activity (both above 90%). Unfortunately, the gender of the partner/perpe-trator was not asked. Muehlenhard and Cook infer that, because most of the men reported being heterosexual and most of the unwanted sex for men was nonviolent, it seems likely that most of their partners were women. However, of the 6.5% of men who experienced unwanted intercourse, it would be particularly important to know who the other person was in these cases, to rule out male perpetrators as well as incestuous abuse by a family member during childhood.

Overall, women reported significantly higher levels of physical coercion to engage in unwanted sexual activity (31%), although almost one-fourth of men also reported this (24%). Most of the unwanted sexual activity resulting from physical coercion was due to nonviolent physical coercion. Violent physical coercion was much less frequent and not significantly different for men and women: Less than 4% of men and women had experienced violent coercion to engage in any unwanted sexual activity, and less than 3% experienced violent coercion to engage in unwanted intercourse. Unfortunately, a breakdown for the physical coercion factor response by gender was not provided, nor were the actual situational contexts in which these experiences occurred. Muehlenhard and Cook note that both nonviolent and violent physical coercion loaded on the same factor for women's data but on different factors for men's data, suggesting that these behaviors are more similar when used against women than when used against men. The most common pressures reported by men were sexual enticement (57%), altruism or a desire to help the woman (35%), and intoxication (31%). The most common reason found for unwanted sex among men appeared to be social pressure related to the male stereotype, including the expectation that men should always want sex and always be ready to perform with an erection (Zilbergeld, 1978).

I contend that, by divorcing this type of research (Muehlenhard & Cook, 1988; Struckman-Johnson, 1988) from the context of power and by applying the inappropriate template of gender neutrality, much information is lost during data collection itself in the selection of variables measured, and much information is later obscured by utilizing categories that hide the real differences in gender and sexual aggression. Measurement that includes context and detailed descriptions would promote more accurate understanding in this area.

There are indeed a small number of men who have been violently sexually assaulted by women, who could not escape, and who are psychologically traumatized by the experience. Due to male sex role expectations that a man should be able to defend himself from women or the belief that a man cannot be raped by a woman, these men may internalize self-blame and have a more difficult time seeking help. The psychological suffering of these men includes many of the same effects observed for female rape victims (Groth & Burgess, 1980; Myers, 1989). However, these cases appear to be among a small minority of men who report experiences of physical coercion, between 1% and 7% (Murphy, 1984; Muehlenhard & Cook, 1988). In these two studies, the type of physical coercion is not indicated. Struckman-Johnson (1991) provides a number of case examples of sexual assault of men by women. The more unusual examples included a man assaulted by a group of women wielding a knife and a man engaged in playful bondage that turned into coerced sex. The more common examples were those in which women used an aggressive but not forceful sexual approach, most often using verbal tactics. Struckman-Johnson and Struckman-Johnson (1994) found that, among the most recent incidents of female-initiated coercion in a sample of 204 men, the most commonly used tactics were persuasion (78%) and intoxication (43%). The least often used tactics were weapons (0%), physical harm (1%), and "scared you with size" (1%). In the two incidents described in which physical pressure was used, both men were able to stop the woman's sexual advance. The arguments presented here are not intended to trivialize the pain of anyone but are concerned with the more typical experiences of sexually coerced men.

## PARALLELS IN RESEARCH ON SEXUAL COERCION AND PARTNER ABUSE

Parallel methodological problems that arise from applying gender neutrality to research on sexual coercion are also problematic in research on partner abuse. Simply measuring the frequency of violent behaviors by men and women does not reveal any gender differences, but questions about the degree of injury, severity of violence, provocation, and motivation for engaging in partner violence reveal significant gender differences. For example, Hamberger and Lohr (1994) found that the two primary factors related to female perpetrators' motivations were self-defense and escape, with retaliation for past violence third, whereas for men, anger expression and domination were the most common. Saunders (1986) questioned women in a battered women's shelter regarding their use of violence, finding that almost 83% reported using at least minor violence at some point in their relationship. However, self-defense or fighting back was the primary reason for the use of violence, whereas other research with men has found that only 5% had used violence for self-defense (Cascardi, Vivian, & Meyer, 1991). Hamberger and Lohr (1994) found no male perpetrators reporting motivations for their violence of self-defense, escape, or retaliation for past physical abuse. Severity of violence was also overlooked initially in the spouse abuse literature. Adler (1981) and Greenblat (1981), both cited in Saunders (1986, pp. 49–50), present interview data that highlight qualitative differences between male and female spousal violence. In some cases, both partners knew that the women's hardest punches did not hurt her partner, and, in fact, the man laughed in response to them. If only quantitative data are considered, however, this would count as "husband abuse." As Andrea Dworkin (1995) wrote, "This [past] research equates a woman's pushing a man away with a man's pushing a woman down a flight of stairs."

## THE REALITY OF VIOLENCE AGAINST WOMEN

Before beginning a discussion of how the term "male rape" has been appropriated and misused by antifeminist backlash proponents, it is important to include a dose of reality on how women fare in our culture with regard to rape and violence. Within this context the critique of backlash ideology can be better understood.

As documented by Goodman, Koss, and Russo (1993), sexual and physical violence against women in the United States is widespread. Nearly six times more women are raped in America than federal statistics indicate, and fewer than one in five ever report the crime to police. A survey sponsored by the National Victim Center and the Crime Victims Research and Treatment Center (1992) found that one in eight women has been the victim of a rape. Women's accounts indicated that more than six of ten rapes are committed against teenagers and young girls, and nearly one-third of all rapes are against girls age eleven or younger. More than 70% of the rape victims knew their attackers well. Thirty-nine percent of rape victims sustain a nongenital physical injury, including abrasions about the head, neck, and face, the extremities, and the trunk region; of these, 54% seek medical treatment (Beebe, 1991).

More severe injuries include multiple traumas, major fractures, and major lacerations (Geist, 1988). Posttrauma skeletal muscle tension is associated with fatigue, tension headaches, and sleep disturbances. Almost one-third of rapes involve oral or anal penetration in addition to vaginal contact, and one-half of rape victims seen in trauma centers have vaginal and perineal trauma (Geist, 1988; Woodling & Kossoris, 1981). Fifteen percent of raped women have significant vaginal tears, and 1% require surgical repair (Cartwright & the Sexual Assault Study Group, 1987). Infection with sexually transmitted diseases (4–30%) and pregnancy (5%) may also result from rape (Goodman et al., 1993). Nearly one in three rape victims develops posttraumatic stress disorder.

Accounts of women's experiences of acquaintance rapes, which represent 70% of women's rapes, must be understood within the social context of violence against women:

> When Sandy's date asked if she minded stopping by his apartment to pick up some papers before having lunch, she told him she didn't mind. But once inside, her date asked her to watch X-rated movies and to kiss him. When she refused, "He grabbed me by the hair . . . twisted my arm behind my back and pushed me back to the bedroom," she said. Sandy ignored his orders to disrobe, but the man ripped off her clothes and forced her to pose before a home-movie camera. "Then he raped me twice," Sandy said about the attack. (Cantwell, 1987, Section A, p. 9)

Attitudes supportive of rape that are held by many men (Burt, 1980; Briere, Malamuth, & Check, 1985) include the belief that if a man becomes sexually aroused on a date, the woman is obligated to provide sex. A student attending the same university as "Sandy" (described above) stated, "They (women) are just saying no, but they're not leaving when a man gets turned on." This rape-supportive belief is expressed clearly by a male writer to columnist Ann Landers (1986): "The problem is that with many men, there is only one way to end arousal and that is ejaculation. At the height of ecstasy, does the female partner think the man is going to excuse himself, go into the bathroom, and take a cold shower? No way. He wants the final act." These are attitudes based on many men's sense of entitlement, backed up in most cases by the physical strength to make good on their threat. The difference between a sexually uninterested man or woman on a date with a sexually desirous partner is that in most cases the man is able to end the sexual interaction and walk away, as noted even in the most "physically violent" case examples described in Struckman-Johnson (1991). For women, this is, realistically, less often an option. For women who are raped by strangers, frequently the most pressing concern is surviving with one's life. Below is such an account:

> "On July 4, 1990, I went for a morning walk along a peaceful-looking country road in southern France. It was a gorgeous day . . . I sang to myself as I set out. . . . An hour later, I was lying near death, pleading for my life with a brutal assailant who had jumped me from behind. I hadn't heard or seen him coming. He dragged me off the road into a deep ravine, beat me with his fist and with a rock, sexually assaulted me, choked me repeatedly and, after I passed out four times, left me for dead." (Brison, 1993, p. 20)

While the accounts of the two women rape victims above are not unusual occurrences for women, both examples would be highly atypical for male victims of female sexual aggression.

## APPROPRIATION OF MALE RAPE BY THE BACKLASH AGAINST FEMINISM

The term "male rape" is potentially very problematic unless great specificity is used to define this term. As with research on domestic violence, research on sexual coercion should assess specific descriptions of the actual behavior, type and severity of physical force used, perceived inability to escape physically, perceived inability to escape psychologically, and degree of threat of physical harm or threat to life experienced. Assessing the gender of both victim and perpetrator is crucial in differentiating the presence of cross-gender from same-gender sexual aggression.

The need for a gender-sensitive analysis requiring much specificity in use of terms and measurement is crucial to avoid misinterpretation and misuse of research findings. For example, Macchietto (1992) cited both Struckman-Johnson's (1988) and Muehlenhard and Cook's (1988) research, arguing that men comprise a significant portion of rape victims: "Thus, when the violent physical coercion category of Muehlenhard and Cook's research is viewed as sexual assault or rape, men make up approximately one-third of the 'rape victims' " (p. 383). Macchietto's misleading extrapolation is possible because of the lack of information regarding the actual circumstances in which violence was used against men in these studies, including the gender of the perpetrator, the degree of restraint or threat used, and the ability to escape the situation. For example, one of the violent-physical-coercion items in Muehlenhard and Cook appears to be, "The other person tried to physically detain you (e.g., he/she blocked your car door to make it difficult to leave, or wouldn't let go of your hand." Another is, "The other person actually used physical violence (e.g., slapping, hitting)." For both of these items, the genders of the victim and perpetrator could imply quite different scenarios and escape options for the victims. It is difficult to imagine many men being physically forced to have sex because a woman wouldn't let go of his hand, although the reverse is more conceivable. However, another item, "The other person threatened you with a weapon," is more likely to be a gender equalizer, as use of a weapon does not depend on physical strength. Placing in the same category men's and women's experiences of violent physical coercion to engage in unwanted sexual activity without a more detailed breakdown of the type of coercion allows for the misleading statement that one-third of victims of violent rape are men. The term "male rape" is a generally misleading description of the typical male experience of sexual coercion by women and carries with it the risk of trivializing and undermining the seriousness of widespread rape of women in our culture.

Equating male rape with women's typical experiences of rape trivializes the more extensive damage, both physical and psychological, to women rape victims. Another attempt to delegitimize women's experiences of rape, particularly acquaintance rape, was launched by Farrell (1993) and has been more recently taken up by Roiphe (1993a) in her construal of the "rape-crisis feminism." Farrell argues, based on Muehlenhard and Cook's (1988) data, that because over 90% of both men and women said that they had unwanted sexual activity by the time they were in college and because 63% of the men and 46% of the women said they had experienced unwanted intercourse, then "by feminist definitions of rape as unwanted sex, virtually everyone has been raped. And that's how rape begins to look like an epidemic. It's also how rape gets trivialized" (Farrell, 1993, p. 317). Farrell does not mention Muehlenhard and Cook's conclusion that the most common reason found for unwanted sex among men appeared to be social pressure related to the male stereotype. Although sequelae of forced-sex incidents were not assessed in Muehlenhard and Cook (1988), Struckman-Johnson (1988) found significantly more negative short- and long-term effects reported by women (88% and 78%) compared to men (27% and 22%). It is crucial to recognize that women are more often traumatized by both physically violent and nonviolent unwanted sexual activity. This is not necessarily because women are more frail psychologically but because gender is not a neutral factor in mediating the experience of sexual coercion. Farrell argues that both men and women have sex when they don't want to and that this is especially true in a relationship, in which both genders engage in "mercy sex": "All good relationships require 'giving in,' especially when our partner feels strongly. The *Ms.* survey can call it a rape; a relationships counselor will call it a relationship" (Farrell, 1993, p. 338). Farrell ridicules the notion of women considering themselves raped if they felt forced and implies that a definition of rape that includes fear or threat, or other forms of coercion short of actual violence, accounts for the increase seen in reported rape. I contend that when women feel forced, within the social context of power inequality and violence in which we live, this may be enough to consider it to be rape in many cases. When men feel compelled to have sex due to peer pressure and a desire to be popular (Muehlenhard & Cook, 1988), or because of a need to live up to the male sexual stereotype, or even because of physical coercion by women, this phenomenon is occurring in an essentially different gender universe. While engaging in unwanted sexual experience is never desirable, these experiences must be understood as different in context and severity of impact.

Roiphe (1993a), a graduate student in English literature, published a book entitled *The Morning After: Sex, Fear, and Feminism on Campus.* This book picks up where Farrell has left off in its attempts to undermine the reality of acquaintance rape on college campuses. Roiphe's thesis is that college activists fighting rape have so exaggerated the dangers that they cause unnecessary terror, blur the distinction between being the victim of a rape and simply having a "bad night," and reawaken old stereotypes of bestial male predators and fragile female victims. Roiphe (1993b) writes in a sarcastic tone about the experiences of victimization shared by women speaking at a "Take Back the Night" rally, rendering her own judgment of the "legitimacy" of the rapes described. Roiphe wants women to take responsibility for their own alcohol consumption, to be outspoken about what they want and don't want, and to see themselves as forceful and lusty. As Roiphe says of her own upbringing, "I was always taught to be strong and assertive and to say what I thought" (cited in Span, 1993, p. L5). Roiphe implies that if a woman does not do these things, then she is responsible for her rape. Perhaps it is Roiphe's relatively privileged and unusual upbringing that blinds her to the prevalence of rape among her peers, and she may not be perceived as a sympathetic audience with whom to share one's rape experience. As Roiphe (1993b) cites herself from *The Morning After,* "If I were really standing in the middle of an epidemic, a crisis, if 25 percent of my female friends were really being raped, wouldn't I know it? (p. 26)." In fact, the best available data on rape in college populations (Koss, Gidycz, & Wisniewski, 1987) found, among a sample of 3,187 college women, that one in four had experienced either rape or attempted rape since age 14, with 15.4% rape and 12.1% attempted-rape survivors. Even when an item that asks, "Have you ever had sexual intercourse when you didn't want to because a man gave you alcohol or drugs?" was excluded, one in five women reported experiencing rape or attempted rape. It may be difficult for a relatively privileged, outspoken, empowered woman like Roiphe to identify with her less assertive and privileged sisters, and her tendency is to blame women who have been victimized in dating situations. However, as Andrea Parrot points out, "Women have less economic power, less political power, less physical power. When you're on a date, the man's paying, the man's deciding where to take you. . . . We can't expect men and women to have an equal opportunity to get out of dangerous situations. That's not the United States in 1993" (Parrot, cited in Span, 1993, p. L5). In fact, Muehlenhard (1988) found that rape-justifiability and sex-willingness ratings were highest when the woman initiated the date, when they went to the man's apartment, and when the man paid the dating expenses. "Men's sex-willingness ratings were consistently higher than women's, suggesting that a man may overestimate his date's interest in sex and may later feel 'led on,' which some males regard as justifying rape" (Muehlenhard,

1988, p. 20). The concern among feminists who research rape and treat its victims is that Roiphe's skepticism emboldens those who have always denied the extent of rape and seen women as its instigators ("She asked for it") or who have made arrest and prosecution difficult and degrading. As Roiphe writes, "There is a gray area in which one person's rape may be another's bad night" (1983b, p. 28). Mary Koss commented, "What Roiphe is doing just breaks my heart. This is already a group of women who don't feel very legitimate, who blame themselves" (Koss, cited in Span, 1993, p. L5).

This debate over the legitimacy of date rape illuminates the basic paradox in attempting to establish consent in the context of asymmetrical power between men and women. As Susan Estrich, a professor of law at the University of Southern California Law Center, writes:

> Many feminists would argue that so long as women are powerless relative to men, viewing a "yes" as a sign of true consent is misguided. . . . For myself, I am quite certain that many women who say yes to men they know, whether on dates or on the job, would say no if they could. I have no doubt that women's silence sometimes is the product not of passion and desire but of pressure and fear. (1987, p. 102)

And as Catharine MacKinnon writes: "Compare victims' reports of rape with women's reports of sex. They look a lot alike. . . . In this light, the major distinction between intercourse (normal) and rape (abnormal) is that the normal happens so often that one cannot get anyone to see anything wrong with it" (cited in Roiphe, 1993, p. 40), Within the context of a patriarchy in which women remain subordinate in status, it is no wonder that defining sexual relations between unequals becomes confusing. This debate about rape should be predicated on an understanding of gender inequality and sexual relations, with the acknowledgment that there is no such thing as gender-neutral experiences of sexual coercion or even of consensual sexual relations within a gender-asymmetric power structure. The most accurate framing of the question about sexual consent would be under what circumstances or to what degree is sexual consent for women possible within a patriarchy? By framing this question not in terms of absolutes (women can never give sexual consent vs. women can always give sexual consent) we can begin to examine to what degree sexual consent is compromised.

## REFERENCES

Adler, E. M. (1981). The underside of married life: Power, influence, and violence. In L. H. Bowker (Ed.), *Women and crime in America* (pp. 300–320). New York: Macmillan.

Beebe, D. (1991). Emergency management of the adult female rape victim. *American Family Physician, 43,* 2041–2046.

Briere, J., Malamuth, N., & Check, J. (1985). Sexuality and rape-supportive beliefs. *International Journal of Women's Studies, 8,* 398–403.

Brison, S. (1993, March 21). Survival course. *New York Times,* Section 6, pp. 20–22.

Burt, M.(1980). Cultural myths and supports for rape. *Journal of Personality and Social Psychology, 38,* 217–230.

Cantwell, G. (1987, May 3). Date-rape studies indicate many assailants are students. *Houston Post,* Section A, p. 9.

Cartwright, P., & The Sexual Assault Study Group. (1987). Factors that correlate with injury sustained by survivors of sexual assault. *Obstetrics and Gynecology, 70,* 44–46.

Cascardi, M., Vivian, D., & Meyer, S. (1991, November). *Context and attributions for marital violence in discordant couples.* Paper presented at the meeting of the Association for Advancement of Behavior Therapy, New York, NY.

Dworkin, A. (1995, July 21). A man's world. *New York Times Book Review,* p. 23.

Estrich, S. (1987). *Real rape: How the legal system victimizes women who say no.* Cambridge, MA: Harvard University Press.

Farrell, W. (1993). *The myth of male power: Why men are the disposable sex.* New York: Simon & Schuster.

Geist, R. (1988). Sexually related trauma. *Emergency Medical Clinics of North America, 6,* 439–466.

Goodman, L., Koss, M., & Russo, N. (1993). Violence against women: Physical and mental health effects. Part I: Research findings. *Applied and Preventive Psychology, 2,* 79–89.

Greenblat, C. (1981, July). *Physical force by any other name. . . . Quantitative data, qualitative data, and the politics of family violence research.* Paper presented at the national Conference for Family Violence Researchers, University of New Hampshire, Durham, NH.

Groth, A. N., & Burgess, A. (1980). Male rape: Offenders and victims. *American Journal of Psychiatry, 137,* 806–810.

Hamberger, L., & Lohr, J. (1994). The intended function of domestic violence is different for arrested male and female perpetrators. *Family Violence and Sexual Assault Bulletin, 10*(3–4), 40–44.

Koss, M., Gidycz, C., & Wisniewski, N. (1987). The scope of rape: Incidence and prevalence of sexual aggression and victimization in a national sample of higher education students. *Journal of Consulting and Clinical Psychology, 55*, 162–170.

Landers, A. (1991, August 4). A male viewpoint on date rape. *Bryan-College Station Eagle,* Section C, p. 3.

Macchietto, J. (1992). Aspects of male victimization and female aggression: Implications for counseling men. *Journal of Mental Health Counseling, 14*(3), 375–392.

Muehlenhard, C. (1988). Misinterpreted dating behaviors and the risk of date rape. *Journal of Social and Clinical Psychology, 6*(1), 20–37.

Muehlenhard, C., & Cook, S. (1988). Men's self-reports of unwanted sexual activity. *Journal of Sex Research, 24*, 58–72.

Murphy, J. (1984, August). *Date abuse and forced intercourse among college students.* Paper presented at the Second National Conference for Family Violence Research, Durham, NH.

Myers, M. (1989). Men sexually assaulted as adults and sexually abused as boys. *Archives of Sexual Behavior, 18*, 203–215.

National Victim Center and the Crime Victims Research and Treatment Center. (1992). *Rape in America: A report to the nation.* Arlington, VA, and Charleston, SC: Author.

O'Sullivan, L., & Byers, E. (1993). Eroding stereotypes: College women's attempts to influence reluctant male sexual partners. *Journal of Sex Research, 30*(3), 270–282.

Roiphe, K. (1993a). *The morning after: Sex, fear, and feminism on campus.* Boston: Little, Brown.

Roiphe, K. (1993b, June 13). Rape hype betrays feminism. *New York Times Magazine,* Section 6, pp. 26, 28, 30, 40, 68.

Sarrel, P., & Masters, W. (1982). Sexual molestation of men by women. *Archives of Sexual Behavior, 11*, 117–131.

Saunders, D. (1986). When battered women use violence: Husband abuse or self defense. *Violence and Victims, 1*, 47–60.

Span, P. (1993, November 14). Date rape: Crisis or hype? *Sunday Oregonian,* Section L, pp. 1, 5.

Struckman-Johnson, C. (1988). Forced sex on dates: It happens to men, too. *Journal of Sex Research, 24*, 234–241.

Struckman-Johnson, C. (1991). Male victims of acquaintance rape. In A. Parrot & L. Bechhofer (Eds.), *Acquaintance rape: The hidden crime* (pp. 192–214). New York: Wiley.

Struckman-Johnson, C., & Struckman-Johnson, D. (1994). Men pressured into forced sexual experience. *Archives of Sexual Behavior, 23*(1), 93–114.

Woodling, B., & Kossoris, P. (1981). Sexual misuse: Rape, molestation, and incest. *Pediatric Clinics of North America, 28,* 481–499.

Working Women's United Institute. (1978). *Responses of fair employment practices agencies to sexual harassment complaints: A report and recommendations.* New York: Working Women's Institute, Research Series Report No. 2.

Zilbergeld, B. (1978). *Male sexuality: A guide to sexual fulfillment.* New York: Little, Brown.

# IV

## TREATMENT AND PREVENTION OF FEMALE SEXUAL AGGRESSION

There is very little known about treatment and prevention programs for receivers and initiators of female sexual aggression. In Chapter 10, John G. Macchietto offers professional advice for counseling men who have been sexually victimized by women. Relating his personal experiences with female verbal sexual aggression, Macchietto explores the concept of "male as victim" and reasons why society has difficulty acknowledging the sexual vulnerability of men.

Andrea Parrot presents in Chapter 11 recommendations for designing programs to prevent the sexual coercion of men. Parrot is one of the leading experts in the country on prevention of acquaintance rape of women on college campuses. In this pioneering chapter, she reviews formats, use of facilitators, activities, and media that can be used in programs for potential male victims and female perpetrators. Parrot includes samples of several exercises that promote student discussion and understanding of factors that contribute to sexual assault.

# 10

## Treatment Issues of Adult Male Victims of Female Sexual Aggression

### JOHN G. MACCHIETTO

Treating men who have been sexually victimized by women is likely to be one of the greatest challenges of a psychotherapist's career. First, there is little research on the topic. A scant body of literature reveals that men make up one-third to 42% of sexually victimized adults (Muehlenhard & Cook, 1988; Struckman-Johnson & Struckman-Johnson, 1994). Even though these estimates suggest that men comprise a fair percentage of sexual victimizations, treatment literature on the subject is extremely scarce. Thus, a psychotherapist's skill at treating male victims of sexually aggressive women is often acquired through trial and error from clinical interactions.

Second, a therapist treating men who have been sexually victimized by women faces barriers to providing that treatment because this concept violates several societal stereotypes. Because of these violated stereotypes, the therapist may fail to perceive that male clients have been victimized or that female clients are perpetrators. Clients may cling to the denial that abuse has occurred. My experience with victimized male clients is that they will present themselves in counseling for other problems and have a difficult time acknowledging their victimization or its relatedness to their presenting problems.

Third, dealing with men who have been sexually victimized by women is considered to be a politically incorrect topic. This makes it very difficult to have an open and healthy dialogue, both for the mental health community and the general public. My own experience is that my discussing or writing about this topic professionally has resulted in a great amount of hostility from several of my peers and other critics who would disagree with me. It has also alienated me from some of my peers, who agree with me, but only privately because they fear being put in a situation where they might become disenfranchised from mainstream thought. This political climate encourages the stereotypes to continue and places a cloak of invisibility over many who would otherwise debate the topic openly. Thus, it interferes with treating both male and female clients who are involved with male victimization by women.

In an earlier article, I outlined what I considered to be five basic treatment techniques or strategies in treating adult men who were victimized sexually or physically by women (Macchietto, 1992). This chapter elaborates on those five strategies. Further, the topic of sexual victimization of men by women will be discussed to establish the theoretical context.

## MEN'S VICTIMIZATION IN CONTEXT

In order to understand men's sexual victimization by women, two areas of context for victimization need to be established: (1) that victimization for men holds negative societal stereotypes and (2) that this topic is considered politically incorrect.

### Victimization Stereotypes of Men and Women

Acknowledging victimization of men by women violates two of society's stereotypes: (1) that women are weak and need protection from men and (2) that men are strong and thus it is unmasculine to be abused by a woman. For therapists to deal effectively with victimized men, they need to develop an appreciation and understanding that the phenomenon exists and that society ignores the reality of men as sexual victims. When these aspects are understood, specific treatment procedures are many and are only limited by a therapist's imagination. To introduce how these stereotypes are entwined, I offer two early personal experiences. When I was in my upper 20s and working on my doctorate at the University of Kansas, I gave a great deal of personal and professional attention to gender issues that were relevant on campus. One such issue was that of the rape of women on campus, and in my role as a men's rights activist, I wanted to understand and articulate how men related to this issue. I was (and am) concerned that rape is a hideous crime. In understanding "rape," however, I was confused by my observation that "rape fantasy" was a popular theme among women's romance novels. I noted that women were angered by the topic of rape while at the same time it was a major theme found in romance novels predominantly read by women. I wanted to discern how a rape fantasy differed from the reality of rape itself. Quite ironically, I had two closely related experiences that helped me to perceive the distinction.

One afternoon, while I was walking across the KU campus, a group of three or four women were on a fire escape of the architecture building yelling sexually aggressive statements at some man. Involved in thought, I did not realize until I was near the building that the unknown women were directing their comments toward me. When I realized they were explicitly commanding me to perform several different sexual acts with them, I became intensely fearful, and I changed my direction to avoid walking by the building by taking a three-block detour. What confused me was that this was the enactment of a consistent fantasy I had as a male: to be desired aggressively by one or a group of women. I was confused at the time that my emotional reaction was quite different.

The next day I was walking to the KU Student Union to attend, ironically enough, a rape prevention program being held by a women's group on campus. I entered the basement area of the student union, and there was a group of about six or seven women in the elevator, holding the door and encouraging me to ride with them. Ignoring my intuition over the "logic" that women could not harm me, I entered the elevator and immediately felt intimidated as the doors shut. I heard one woman's voice saying I had a "cute little butt" and another commenting on how she liked my shoulders. There were other similar comments, but my attention turned to a hand that began touching my back, another that touched my left arm and another that began to massage my buttocks. The door opened unexpectedly on the third floor to pick up another passenger, and I darted out to climb the steps to my fifth-floor destination. As with my earlier experience, I was very confused at how fearful I felt over an event I had recently fantasized about so positively. My conclusion was that "rape fantasies" were not really rape fantasies but rather "disguised seduction fantasies."

In my fantasy life, I visualized a rape scenario so that I could be "seduced" in sexual excitement without the guilt of being a willing participant or having the task of being the initiator so perennial of the male role. The fear and disgust I had with those two experiences occurred because the actual experience of being overpowered by others was *not* seduction but that of a "rape" mentality, and I was experiencing this aggression by women. For me, this helped explain why women in our society can hold a rape fantasy so strongly in the media of romance and simultaneously be vehemently opposed to a "rape culture." I reasoned that men were really no different and that *people* often confused the line that separates rape/seduction fantasies from rape itself.

Perhaps the most profound learning I had with these experiences was that, when I did begin to tell my men and women friends, I was greeted with considerable laughter, in a tone that indicated I was not to be taken seriously. The most common comment I received was that I must have "really enjoyed it." It bothered me more that these comments were being made by my counseling peers and others who were "knowledgeable" in gender issues and that there seemed to be no difference in attitudes between my male and female peers—people who I felt should have known better. People who were very aware that it would be insensitive and vulgar to tell a woman that she must have enjoyed aggressive men on an elevator had a different attitude toward me as a man in a circumstance that was identical except for the fact that the gender roles were reversed. When confronted with this discrepancy, my peers persisted "jokingly" that I was overreacting because men enjoy and welcome this sort of sexual advance and that most men would be envious. After all, I was a man. It was only in a few men's support groups that my discussing this was taken seriously and by men who were articulate in understanding "men's issues." I also learned that several of the men in these groups had also had similar experiences in their lives but, like myself, dismissed their feelings at the time because of their sense of ridicule over the incidents.

This led me to question why there was so much resistance to *male* victimization, particularly when the victimization was sexual. The little research on the topic is in itself evidence of the resistance. Over several years, I have developed a list of what I believe to be the predominant reasons why this resistance exists. To understand this, it is important to examine the concept of victimization in relationship to masculinity. Men have been raised to be protectors of women. Male chivalry is the action reflecting the attitude that women need protection from other men. However, recently male chivalry and protective behavior have been viewed almost exclusively in terms of being chauvinistic or degrading to women. For example, the protective attitude can be seen as a major component of resistance toward women entering the protective services, such as firefighting, police work, and the military. These protective domains have been viewed as "male dominated" areas of work, and women who challenged these stereotypes by entering male protective services have been accused of being "masculine" women. The often-overlooked corollary to this stereotype is that men who need protection themselves, who are not good protectors, are viewed as less masculine or "wimpish." For men to be victimized themselves, or to be viewed as victims, is to be seen as less masculine by a society that holds this stereotype. It makes sense that men, because of their socialization, would resist being viewed as victims, with the help-lessness and emasculation connotations that go along with it. My own experiences with my peers' refusal to see me as violated by aggressive women very effectively tempered my comments to them and motivated me to downplay and ignore my own feelings.

As a present-day nonsexual example, men in our society are routinely ridiculed in the media as people who do not seek directions when lost in a strange city. I have not yet found a comedian or journalist who discusses or questions why so many men seem to resist asking for directions. In view of the tremendous social pressure for men to be in charge and good protectors, looking for directions in a city is a sign that they are somehow not self-sufficient enough to solve the problem. Farrell (1986) discusses at length how men are socialized to be self-sufficient.

Asking for directions is not the only area in which men seem to resist looking non-self-sufficient. For example, the Bureau of Justice Statistics of the U.S. Department of Justice (1995) estimates that, though men are the victims of violent crime approximately twice as often as women, men consistently report crime less frequently than do women. Further, men succeed at suicide four times as often as women and constitute approximately 75% of those hospitalized for alcohol and drug addiction (Farrell, 1993). Although men are more likely than women to die from stress-related diseases, they are less likely to visit physicians for physical symptoms that could be triggered by stress.

Rather than just to observe that men resist asking for directions or to criticize them for this tendency, it is more pragmatic to question why there is a tremendous societal resistance to viewing men as victims. In a clinical setting, to continue to view men's victimization with less credibility than that of women encourages our male and female clients to do likewise. The reluctance of clients (male or female) to view their experience as victimization might best be labeled "denial." Perhaps the best clinical technique to help men through their victimization is to find ways to break down this denial, with clients as well as among therapists.

## Political Incorrectness

I now wish to establish the importance of understanding that the topic of male victimization is considered to be a politically incorrect one. The men's movement itself has had great difficulty in establishing a forum in the media and, consequently, is often misperceived either as being antiwoman or as a group of men who beat drums in the woods in search of their manhood. While I cannot speak for all men, I have been involved as a leader in men's gender issues since 1980 and have been active in a men's activist organization, the National Coalition of Free Men (NCFM), for more than 10 years.

Williamson (1985) wrote a historical perspective of the men's movement from the 1950s to 1985. In it, he identified three basic fragments of the men's movement. One faction was called the "feminist men's movement," which developed in academic circles of men who were sympathetic to their feminist women colleagues; it became a group that greatly criticized men's sexist behavior, chiefly ignoring the context of how that behavior was interrelated to women's sexist behavior. This faction can still be seen in many of the academic organizations in the country. The second faction was called the "quiet movement" and represented groups of men, not collecting out of a political agenda but bonding for support, that did not get much attention. This group today can be seen as the "mythopoetic men's movement" that was popularized in the media in the early 1990s by Robert Bly (1990), who wrote the book *Iron John* and who is known for his drumming groups for men. The third faction was labeled by Williamson as the "nonfeminist men's movement" that grew out of the frustration some men felt over not taking the "guilty" perspective the feminist men's movement espoused and/or not being active or outspoken, as the quiet men's movement endorsed. This faction sought to address men's issues that urged gender equality without apologizing for one's maleness or necessarily agreeing with feminists' view of the world.

With that background, it is understandable that many view the men's movement from a feminist men's perspective; that men articulating how society has been unfair to them is seen as frivolous, "whiny," or minuscule in contrast to women's oppression. However, this feminist perspective is strongly ingrained in our society, and only recently a few authors have made inroads to the general public with a nonfeminist perspective. Warren Farrell's (1993) book, *The Myth of Male Power,* challenges many traditional stereotypes of men and women. Christina Hoff Sommers (1994), in her book *Who Stole Feminism?,* makes a distinction between a "true feminist," who wants equality between men and women, and a "gender feminist," who wants advantage over men. In her opening preface she writes:

American feminism is currently dominated by a group of women who seek to persuade the public that American women are not the free creatures we think we are. The leaders and theorists of the women's movement believe that our society is best described as a patriarchy, a "male hegemony," a "sex/gender system" in which the dominant gender works to keep women cowering and submissive. . . .

The women currently manning—womaning—the feminist ramparts do not take well to criticism. How could they? As they see it, they are dealing with a massive epidemic of male atrocity and a constituency of benighted women who have yet to comprehend the seriousness of their predicament. Hence, male critics must be "sexist" and "reactionary," and female critics "traitors," "collaborators," or "backlashers." This kind of reaction has had a powerful inhibiting effect. It has alienated and silenced women and men alike. (Hoff Sommers, 1994, pp. 16–18)

Hoff Sommers expertly presents several examples of how gender feminists have politically maneuvered and have distorted research to advance their cause. Her book also describes what happens to people who break a stereotype. Men and women alike who become politically incorrect violate the stereotypes that men are strong and that it is unmasculine to be victimized by a woman and that women are weak and need protection from men. In violating this stereotype, men become negatively viewed as "victimized men," and women who can define other women as victimizers are negatively viewed as unworthy to be accepted within the "sisterhood" of good women who advance the cause of feminism.

## Sexual Attitudes

To add to the complexity of men's reluctance to acknowledge sexual victimization, there are a few basic stereotypes surrounding sexuality in our society that need to be addressed. Generally, American culture espouses that sex is bad, wrong, and vulgar. We still refer to sexually oriented jokes as "dirty" jokes. Differences between men and women in experiences regarding sexual expressiveness also exist. For instance, men are taught: (1) that although sex is vulgar, it is their job to initiate sexual activity (men still greatly outnumber women in initiating first dates) and (2) that not to pursue women is considered unmanly ("wimpish," "sissyish," "boring," etc.). *In short, to be sexually expressive (assertive) is part of the societal definition of masculinity.*

In contrast, (1) women are taught that sex is bad and a woman's job is to be pure and resist men's advances (there is great contempt for women who are sexually promiscuous; Stubbs, 1994); and (2) women therefore adapt by acting coy, sexually passive, receptive, and seductive to express their sexuality. *In short, to not be sexually expressive (assertive) is part of the societal definition of femininity.*

Thus, when a woman acts sexually aggressive with a man, social rules and expectations are violated concerning both men and women. The woman is seen as "nonfeminine," and/or the man is seen as "nonmasculine." A sexually violated man must overcome two socially violated rules concerning masculinity: that he is not a self-sufficient man and that he is inept sexually. To add to this conflict, if the man is strong enough himself to recognize that he was violated, then he must next contend with a society that "unjustly" labels him as being less than masculine. Further myths surround the area of female sexual violence. As noted earlier, I experienced a great deal of resistance from my peers when I described how I was sexually harassed by two different groups of women. Further, when I speak publicly about sexual victimization of men to college classes and to other community groups, I routinely spend time explaining the mechanics of "how a man could be raped by a woman." The greatest hurdle seems to be the myth that it would be impossible for a man to achieve or maintain an erection when threatened by a woman; that, somehow, for a man to have an erection means he was enjoying the experience. Sarrel and Masters (1982) noted the stereotype "that it would be almost impossible for a man to achieve or maintain an erection when threatened or attacked by a woman. Widespread acceptance of this sexual myth has unfortunate implications for medicine, psychology and law" (p. 118). They further state that "most women lubricate and some women respond at orgasmic levels while they are being sexually molested" (Sarrel & Masters, 1982, p. 118).

When this myth surfaces, I then present information about sexual responses that both men and women exhibit in relationship to fear. This information has great importance in understanding that men, like women, can be sexual victims as well as perpetrators. The belief that a female sexual assault victim must not be a victim because "she enjoyed it or would not have lubricated" has confused many in society, including those sexually assaulted. Extending this knowledge, just because a man became aroused or even ejaculated when assaulted does not mean he "enjoyed it." This is a necessary step in understanding sexual assault of men. Again, this represents the same confusion I addressed earlier, when I learned to differentiate between a rape and a seduction fantasy.

Another example that demonstrates society's resistance to male victims and female aggressors has to do with date rape where alcohol is a factor. I have discussed date rape in several university classes over the last decade. Inevitably the discussion gravitates to how the laws in most states recognize that a rape occurs when a consensual participant is intoxicated at the time of the sexual contact if that participant recognizes that *she* would not have engaged in the sexual activity if sober. Students are quick to recognize that when a woman has been drinking, her judgment is affected, and, consequently, she may act sexually against her sober judgment. The fact is that most men who are sexual with women who have been drinking have also been drinking themselves. Therefore, to be fair and consistent, those men can logically claim that they were date raped themselves if they believe they were sexually active against their sober judgment. When bringing this point up to student groups, I inevitably get a great deal of initial shock. However, most students that I have presented this information to quickly recognize their previous inconsistency in logic and agree that men, like women, can and are raped when this definition is consistent for both genders. Discussing this allows a clearer understanding of the double standard that exists in society that says that nonsober women are raped, whereas intoxicated men are rapists. It is important to note that this double standard is consistent with believing that men are the sexual aggressors/initiators and women are sexually helpless or passive.

## TREATMENT TECHNIQUES

With this in mind, the described five techniques to treat men who have been sexually victimized by women will be clearer. This is not an exhaustive list, but it does serve to provide those in the mental health field with a foundation for understanding how to proceed in helping men therapeutically with their victimization. These techniques are (1) recognition; (2) role reversal; (3) stereotype busting; (4) direct reframing; and (5) universal education.

### Recognition

Recognition is an overall awareness of victimization in its many subtle forms. Society's stereotypes strongly affect how and who we view to be victims and/or aggressors. As discussed, men who are victimized must deal with not only their victimization but also with assimilating victimization into their lives in a society that defines victimization as being nonmasculine. Consequently, a technique that is effective in changing a stereotype first makes the stereotype visible. In other words, one important way to recognize stereotypes is to learn as much as one can about the common stereotypes. As most feminists know, just being a woman does not mean one is knowledgeable in women's issues. There are many aspects to be learned about women's oppression that have been discussed and articulated over the last three decades by contemporary feminism. The same is true for understanding men's issues. Just being male does not make one articulate and knowledgeable about men's issues.

An early feminist, Jane O'Reilly, became famous among feminists for defining a phenomenon she coined as a "click." A click was a recognition of incongruity when a women first notices sexism in its subtle form. In other words, when a woman first recognizes that her opinions are not valued in the workplace because she is a woman she has a "click" experience. Society has had three decades of feminism articulating and publicizing click experiences of women in all forms of media. Society has not had a strong men's movement with the same media coverage that has articulated many of the male click experiences. Consequently, society has a much stronger understanding of sexism against women. A men's rights activist might ask (and these are just a few questions), "If men are so favored in our society, why do they die seven years before women?" "Why do recently single men commit suicide eleven times more often than recently single women?" "Why are 85% of the homeless men?" If women died seven years before their male peers, if they committed suicide eleven times more often than men when they became single, if they made up 85% of the homeless, do you think it would be unnoticed in the media today? Rather, you would likely see news coverage and special reports on "early *female* death," "*women's* suicide," and the "*female* homeless" problem. You would also find several commentaries on how these situations are clear examples of a patriarchy and women's oppression in society.

In contrast, there is little coverage in the media about male click experiences. A click experience implies an injustice and/or victimization. It makes sense in a society that considers male victimization unmasculine that those "click" experiences would not be viewed as clicks. This is consistent with my peers viewing my encounters with sexually harassing women as being a stroke of luck instead of harassment. Therapists, then, who wish to become knowledgeable of male click experiences will need to look diligently with that goal in mind and not accept the feminist perspective of what men's issues are or what they should be. To ask feminists to define men's issues would be akin to expecting early feminists to go to the "patriarchal leaders" of their times to understand and define women's issues. Instead, women leaders communicated among themselves and began to articulate a new understanding of the experience of being a woman in our society. To do the same for understanding men's issues, it is crucial for therapists to recognize the stereotypes that constrict men.

Since the men's movement has not had the same articulation in the media as the women's movement, therapists wanting to understand men's issues may conceivably have some trouble in locating sources. Fortunately, there are a few good sources that concisely articulate men's issues that have made their way into the mass media. Christina Hoff Sommers's (1994) book, *Who Stole Feminism?*, and Warren Farrell's (1993) book, *The Myth of Male Power*, are two strong sources that identify stereotypes of men. Other noteworthy books are Francis Baumli's (1985) *Men Freeing Men*, Susan Jeffers's (1989) *Opening Our Hearts to Men*, Jack Kammer's (1994) *Good Will toward Men*, and Farrell's (1986) *Why Men Are the Way They Are.*

These sources are a place for therapists to become aware of what stereotypes exist that limit men. While a therapist need not agree with all or any of what these authors present, the stereotypes will become visible, and thus the first step in addressing the stereotypes that limit their clients' lives will be taken.


## Role Reversal

With an understanding that men are sexually victimized by women, role reversal as a technique becomes quite simple. Therapists conceptualize reversing the sex of the client to help make male victims and female aggressors visible to both clients and therapists. For example, while counseling a 19-year-old male student who was having sexual adjustment problems with his fiancée of 1 year, I conceptualized what I would ask him if he were a woman presenting the same situation. I reasoned that a woman with this presenting problem would likely be dealing with general societal repression of her sexuality or pressure from her fiancé to engage in sex or that she may be a victim of sexual abuse.

With my male client, then, I proceeded to explore the same three hypotheses I would have asked with a hypothetical female client. My male client seemed very nervous about his sexual history. Using the described recognition strategy, I asked him how old he was when he had his first sexual experience. Eventually, he described an event that occurred when he was 15 years old. He explained *he* was sexual with his sister's 19- or 20-year-old female friend. He initially presented the incident as one in which he was a willing participant and inferred that he initiated the experience. However, when asked to clarify what specifically had happened, it became obvious to both of us that she initiated and controlled the sexual encounter very aggressively. He expressed his fear, shame, and reluctance to engage in genital petting and intercourse with her but said he did so on the threat that she would tell his sister "*he* attacked her" if he did not comply with her demands. Consistent with Sarrel and Masters's (1982) description, he detailed his belief that he was not victimized because he maintained an erection during intercourse and even ejaculated.

## Stereotype Busting

I chose the term "stereotype busting" to portray a direct attack on the traditional stereotypes held by clients. A skilled therapist can challenge a client's stereotypes by being very direct or very subtle in presentation. For example, if a client refers to a sexual molester with the male pronoun, "he," the therapist can say in a direct approach, "I noticed that you referred to the molester as a male. Perhaps we can discuss this viewpoint." The therapist can also take a less direct approach by paraphrasing the client's response while adding a gender-inclusive reference. For instance, the therapist can say, "So you're fearful that your child may have been molested recently. Do you have any ideas who he or she might be?"

This can be extended to several other gender-inclusive references in other areas of victimization. The most frequent response I receive from women listening to my acknowledgment of "husband abuse" is one of initial puzzlement, then reflection; then they provide examples of men they know who have been or are being abused. I have found asking if the client was ever abused by his/her "aunt *or* uncle," "mother *or* father," or "brother *or* sister" to be simple and effective.

This acknowledgment of women's potential for aggression is a display of acceptance, empathy, and respect for female clients, because it says to the client, "If you have a problem losing control and hurting the people you love, I am open to discuss this with you." Credibility builds when therapists are able to confront their clients' issues directly and honestly, no matter what those issues are. For abusive women and victimized men, using clients' gender-specific references inadvertently conveys the attitude that the therapist is either unable, reluctant, or unknowledgeable to discuss their issues or that these clients are very different and abnormal compared to other clients.

## Direct Reframing

Reframing has received considerable attention in psychotherapy as a technique. Basically, reframing presents a new viewpoint of the same facts or situation. Once this is done, a client has a broader perspective of his or her situation, and this allows more options and flexibility for different feelings, attitudes, and behaviors.

There are countless examples of reframing that can be presented here. However, it is pragmatic to highlight a few common patterns and strategies. One strategy I have found to be extremely effective is *explaining* a sex role reversal in detail to clients. First, a therapist acquires as much information as possible about an event, then reverses the sexes in the scenario hypothetically *for the client*. This technique is different from the previously described role reversal technique because the role reversal is communicated directly to the client rather than being used only by a therapist in conceptualizing a strategy.

A clear example of this technique was used with the male client described earlier who was sexually assaulted by his sister's girlfriend. I eventually said to him, "You know, you have told me with great reluctance about her demanding that you have sex with her and that you were scared and frightened. And while your body performed, you were both excited and confused. If you were a female client telling me this, I think I, and most anyone else (and I think even you, too), would call you a rape victim . . . and I know it's not easy to say that because most of society does not recognize sexual assault against men by women, and in many states it is not even legally defined as sexual assault, but it does occur as I think you know" (Macchietto, 1992, p. 387). This client responded well to these remarks. He immediately showed a strong facial expression of relief and later indicated that it was that statement that marked a change in his feeling burdened with that incident.

Another reframing strategy that I have found particularly effective is asking clients their opinions about a movie that portrays a 15-year-old girl who emotionally becomes a woman by having sex with a man in his 30s. Clients are very quick to recognize how this is an exploitive situation of the girl and how this is also considered statutory rape. I then point out that when the genders are reversed to a woman in her 30s having sex with a 15-year-old boy, the movie is called *The Summer of '42,* which was acclaimed as a "romance" movie.

## Universal Education (or the "Other" Sex vs. the "Opposite" Sex)

Universal education is an attempt to provide an understanding to clients that victimization and aggression are universal across sexes. I view this educative goal as paramount in working therapeutically with clients on gender relationship issues. This is because the premise that men and women are more alike than they are different promotes a greater understanding and appreciation of the other sex. In fact, I specifically use the term "the other sex" as opposed to "the opposite sex" to promote the very assumption that men and women are more alike than they are different. When the term "opposite sex" is used, it promotes the polarizing belief that if women are victims, then men must be the opposite, or perpetrators. This is very restrictive thinking, and therapists are wise to maintain that men and women, while they may have different styles and socialization patterns, are still both ultimately human, with the potential for love and hate, compassion and violence, fear and accomplishment, and all the other "human" characteristics.

There is also a pragmatic reason for using universal education. When people see themselves as more alike than different, there is a lesser tendency to feel guilty or to accuse and blame others. Marriage and family therapists know that there is a large amount of guilt and/or blaming within couples who need a great deal of attention and healing. It only makes sense that therapists espouse a value and technique that will aid in healing the guilt and blame.

When the polarizing belief of the "opposite sex" is used, then human characteristics also become polarized by sex. Using universal education helps male clients experience being emotionally vulnerable and compassionate, as women are perceived to be, *in addition* to men's perceived male qualities. This helps men achieve a balance or state of androgyny. Universal education helps women view themselves as powerful, forceful, and aggressive, as men are perceived to be, *in addition* to women's perceived female qualities. This, too, encourages balance for women.

Universal education also provides greater compassion and understanding between the sexes. Men who view vulnerability as a weakness and polarize that trait to women can and do blame women for having that quality. However, when men recognize that same sense of vulnerability in themselves, it is harder to blame women for that trait. Men eventually learn that vulnerability is not a weakness but a strength when used constructively. Likewise, women who view aggression as a weakness and polarize that trait to men can and do blame men. However, when women recognize that same aggressiveness in themselves, it becomes harder to blame men. Women eventually learn that aggressiveness is not necessarily a weakness but can be a strength when used constructively.

To be specific as to how to use the universal education technique in therapy, I offer the following example regarding sexually violated male clients. Presenting specific information about the physiological processes associated with the sexual response to rape provides the understanding that men and women are more alike than different. Sarrel and Masters (1982) observed that of the 11 case examples of men who were sexually abused by women, "a feeling that was prevalent among the men was the sense that they had responded sexually in circumstances in which a normal man would have been impotent. As a result, they came to regard themselves as abnormal, which in turn kindled or rekindled feelings of inadequacy as a man, homosexual anxieties, and sexual performance anxieties" (p. 127).

To explain to male clients who have this problem that it is

*normal* for both men and women to be sexually aroused while frightened and while being raped can help them reduce their anxieties about being "abnormal." It can also help relieve them of any guilt associated with their assuming that they wanted to be raped because they appeared to have "enjoyed it." This very information about sexual arousal is helpful for female sexual abuse victims as well. When both men's and women's physiological processes are discussed, clients can view their responses as normal across people and not just applicable to one sex. Explaining that their responses are universal to *all* human beings increases the chance that their sense of isolation and abnormality will be reduced. This also provides one other clear example of how men and women, who most think are quite different when it comes to being rape victims, actually share common physiological responses. This leads the way for other traits, originally viewed as polarized, to be viewed from a more balanced perspective.

## CONCLUDING REMARKS

In conclusion, I ask, if you found yourself becoming emotionally appalled and irritated or even elated and joyful while reading this chapter, that you reserve judgment until you have introspected on your feelings and how they relate to the contents of this material. Ask yourself if you are reacting more from the logic of what I have written or from the fact that perhaps your own stereotypes have been challenged.

The position I have taken in this chapter is that men and women can both be sexual victims and sexual aggressors. This in itself conflicts with our traditional stereotypes that girls are made of "sugar and spice and everything nice," while boys are made of "snips and snails and puppy dog tails." Stereotypes are usually most invisible to those who hold them. If you have reacted emotionally to this chapter, I am pleased. It means that you have listened to a viewpoint that has challenged your view of the world. This is the first step in clarifying your own beliefs and values. People have more freedom in life when they operate from a clearer understanding of who they are and of their values and belief systems. As therapists, it is necessary that we model flexibility in thinking for our clients.

## REFERENCES

Baumli, F. (1985). *Men freeing men: Exploding the myth of the traditional male.* Jersey City, NJ: New Atlantis Press.

Bly, R. (1990). *Iron John: A book about men.* Reading, MA: Addison-Wesley.

Farrell, W. (1986). *Why men are the way they are: The male–female dynamic.* New York: McGraw-Hill.

Farrell, W. (1993). *The myth of male power: Why men are the disposable sex.* New York: Simon & Schuster.

Hoff Sommers, C. (1994). *Who stole feminism?: How women have betrayed women.* New York: Simon & Schuster.

Jeffers, S. (1989). *Opening our hearts to men.* New York: Fawcett Columbine.

Kammer, J. (1994). *Good will toward men: Women talk candidly about the balance of power between the sexes.* New York: St. Martin's Press.

Macchietto, J. (1992). Aspects of male victimization and female aggression: Implications for counseling men. *Journal of Mental Health Counseling, 14*(3), 375–392.

Muehlenhard, C., & Cook, S. (1988). Men's self-reports of unwanted sexual activity. *Journal of Sex Research, 24,* 58–72.

Sarrel, P., & Masters, W. (1982). Sexual molestation of men by women. *Archives of Sexual Behavior, 11,* 117–131.

Struckman-Johnson, C., & Struckman-Johnson, D. (1994). Men pressured and forced into sexual experience. *Archives of Sexual Behavior, 23,* 93–114.

Stubbs, K. (1994). *Women of the light: The new sacred prostitute.* Larkspur, CA: Secret Garden.

U.S. Department of Justice, Bureau of Justice Statistics. (1995). *Sourcebook of criminal justice statistics, 1994* (Publication No. NCJ-154591). Washington, DC: U.S. Government Printing Office.

Williamson, T. (1985). A history of the men's movement. In F. Baumli (Ed.), *Men freeing men: Exploring the myth of the traditional male* (pp. 308–324). Jersey City, NJ: New Atlantis Press.

# 11

# Meaningful Sexual Assault Prevention Programs for Men

## ANDREA PARROT

Rape does not occur in all cultures; it is a learned behavior. cross-cultural research reveals that rape is absent from certain societies and rampant and ritualized in others (Sanday, 1990). Unfortunately, most normative cultures in the United States condone sexual violence and sexual harassment in both subtle and overt ways that result in men, as well as women, being victimized. In one study, almost two-thirds of college men reported engaging in sex when they did not want to because of peer pressure by other males or wanting to be popular (Muehlenhard & Cook, 1988). Aizenman and Kelley (1988) reported similar findings in their study, in which 14% of male students reported having been forced to have sexual intercourse against their will and 17% of male respondents reported being forced to engage in other forms of unwanted sexual behavior.

While men are being sexually victimized much less often than women, male victimization does happen. The FBI estimates that 10% of all sexual assault victims are men. Men who are at risk for sexual assault victimization are likely to lack assertiveness and are prone to respond to peer pressure. These men probably lack skills to assess situations that can become potentially dangerous. They cannot read the "danger signs" that suggest that the people they are with are likely to disregard their wishes. Men who are sexually victimized are typically assaulted at the hands of a peer, coworker, authority figure, date, or lover rather than by a stranger (Myers, 1989). Men are most often sexually victimized in their teens or early 20s at parties or bars, seduced by trusted individuals (e.g., physicians, psychotherapists, priests, or teachers), or gang raped in military settings or prison by their contemporaries (Goyer & Eddleman, 1984; Groth & Burgess, 1980; Kaufman, Divasto, Jackson, Voorhees, & Christy, 1980; Myers, 1989). The circumstances that lead to sexual assault may include homophobia (in which men often sexually assault other men), alcohol or drug abuse, or a situation in which men are confined, such as prison. Therefore, effective programs for preventing sexual assault of men should begin in the teen years.

## MEN FORCING MEN

Male sexual victimization often occurs within groups that abuse alcohol or drugs. Men are at greatest risk for sexual assault victimization by men who are homophobic and who get caught up in "groupthink." These men may want to punish someone that they believe is homosexual for his sexual orientation by sexually assaulting him orally or anally. Gay men are at some risk of sexual assault by their gay partners (Hickson et al., 1994; Waterman, Dawson, & Bologna, 1989).

## WOMEN FORCING MEN

The belief that men cannot be sexually victimized by women is called the "Myth of Sexual Invulnerability" (Rosenfeld, 1982; Sarrel & Masters, 1982). There is a widely held belief that men are more sexually assertive, sexually oriented, and interested in sex than women (Brehm, 1985; Allgeier & McCormick, 1983). And when women interact with men sexually, women are expected to influence men to avoid sex, not have sex (Clark & Hatfield, 1989). Perhaps because of their lack of experience in coercing others sexually, most women who attempt to do so have little success (O'Sullivan & Byers, 1993). However, some women are successful, and it is those interactions that will be the basis of the majority of the remainder of this chapter.

Men are sexually assaulted by women in situations where alcohol is likely to reduce the inhibitions of the woman and in which the man lacks the self-confidence and self-esteem to leave the situation. Internal pressures a man may experience that leads him to have unwanted sex include the worry that the woman will think either that he is gay or that she lacks sex appeal (Komarovsky, 1976; Weis & Borges, 1973); the fear that he is not a real man because "real men" would never refuse advances by a woman (Doyle, 1983; Zilbergeld, 1978); or his shame at being a virgin (Komarovsky, 1976). In these situations, the woman may hold some power over the man, and he does not feel that he has the choice to avoid the sexual encounter. Men who are sexually assaulted by women report that women use the following strategies (in descending order) to get them to comply: verbal pressure (pleading, coercion, and blackmail), a combination of verbal pressure and physical constraint, excessive intoxication, and physical coercion (Struckman-Johnson, 1991).

## RESPONSIBILITY FOR THE ASSAULT

Sexual assault victims need to understand that the responsibility for rape lies with the perpetrator, regardless of the circumstances of the assault. While peers may coerce others into committing a crime, a victim of a crime *cannot make* the perpetrator commit that crime. Some circumstances can increase the risk of acquaintance rape or sexual assault occurring. Insensitivity to others' feelings, ambiguous sexual norms, differing personal expectations, alcohol use, and peer pressure can interact and contribute to sexual assault.

## PREVENTION STRATEGIES

### Techniques to Educate Men in Avoiding Sexual Assault Victimization

Rape education for men and women can occur in two basic ways: through direct individual educational efforts and by peer pressure. A group's opinion is very effective in establishing normative behavior and is likely to change individual attitudes and behaviors. The most effective rape prevention programs that effectively change behaviors are those that can reach the participants on the cognitive and affective levels.

The strategies necessary for helping men prevent sexual assault victimization differ depending on the circumstances. Sexual assaults of men by other men in prison situations is an extremely complex societal situation, and one well beyond the scope of this chapter. A total revision of the criminal justice system in the United States would be necessary to eliminate or effectively reduce male sexual assault in prisons.

Skills men need to learn to reduce their risk of male sexual assault victimization within the nonprison population include (1) being able to assess situations that are potentially dangerous (e.g., identifying people who abuse power or use alcohol excessively, etc.,), (2) assertiveness, and (3) improving their self-esteem. Improving self-esteem requires a large number of consistently positive experiences and is not likely to be accomplished within only one program. However, a program on sexual assault prevention is a good place to begin this process. People have to respect themselves enough so that they will be less concerned with how their peer group views them. The better their self-esteem, the less likely they are to become victims of sexual assault.

Sexual victimization sometimes occurs because a person is in the wrong place at the wrong time. Potential victims need to be able to assess situations that are potentially dangerous and avoid those situations. Therefore, program participants need to be helped to identify which variables make a situation dangerous (such as intoxicated people, isolated areas, or motives involving exploitation, racism, prejudice, violence, or abuse of power).

Sexual assault of men involves many of the same circumstances and variables are present in the sexual assault of women. Therefore, many of the strategies used for sexual assault prevention for women are also applicable to men. However, the examples used in a presentation aimed at male victims must be adjusted to be appropriate for the target audience.

## Elements Necessary for Prevention Programs for Women Who Are Potential Aggressors

Women who are potential aggressors can overcome their capacity to hurt others by understanding how they become involved in violent behaviors. The continuum of violence might have started in child-hood through modeling adult behavior. It may also be a reaction to the physical, emotional, or sexual abuse they received as children. Some women use physical, psychological, or sexual violence within a specific relationship because of the dynamics of the interaction between them and particular partners. Sometimes this behavior is retaliatory, and at other times it is initiated by women for other reasons. Whatever the reasons, understanding that any kind of violence is the result of a process that was learned and can be unlearned is a good beginning. Another important cognitive reali-zation is that in many states gender-neutral laws allow women, as well as men, to be prosecuted for sexual crimes, including rape.

If women who are likely perpetrators can be helped to empa-thize with their potential victims and the emotional trauma of victimization, they will be less likely to act out their aggression. Some of the information available from other authors in this text who speak about the impact of sexual aggression on men and the confusion, conflict, and fear that men feel about interpersonal relationships may be helpful. In addition, techniques that help women draw on their own past experiences of helplessness, fear, confusion, frustration, and/or violation can promote an atmosphere of care and understanding toward men in place of what might currently be an adversarial one.

Skilled facilitators are a must for dealing with this population. They will be able to create an atmosphere of trust and openness and to promote discussion. Possible triggers for discussion could be clips from movies like *Disclosure* and *Thelma and Louise*.

## Rape Education Strategies for Working With Male, Female, or Mixed Groups

The material presented in this section is based on ideas and materials that should be theoretically effective. However, every group is different, and what may work for one group may fail with another group. In addition, it will be difficult to get men to voluntarily attend a program on how men can avoid sexual assault victimization because most people in this culture believe that only women are victims of sexual assault.

Programs are likely to get best attendance if they are presented where men and women already congregate, such as residence halls, classes, sports teams, sororities/fraternities, and clubs. However, if we take programs to already existing all-male or all-female groups, there will be a mix of types of participants: Some will be potential perpetrators of sexual assault, some will never be involved in sexual assaults as either victims or assailants, and some will be past or future sexual assault victims. Thus, the material should be presented in a manner that allows all the participants to learn effective strategies for preventing sexual assault and assault victimization that they may apply to themselves or share with significant others in their lives (such as siblings, lovers, or friends). In this way, material could be presented for any potential sexual assault victim, regardless of gender. In the beginning of the program, the facilitators must make it clear that both men *and* women are perpetrators as well as victims of sexual assault and that male sexual assault does not only happen in prisons. Therefore, the participants should listen to the information presented and share it with others or use it themselves if it seems appropriate.

## Repeating the Message

A one-time program is likely to have limited success. The more often men and women receive the message in a variety of different ways from a variety of different sources, the more likely it will be to make a lasting impact.

## Programming Based on Theories

Programming should be based on moral development theories. Most successful programs take into account the levels of moral development of the group members. At a typical rape prevention program, there will be men and women at various stages of moral development. William Perry (1970) suggests that college students fall into three basic stages of development: Dualism (right and wrong), Relativism (absolutes may be questioned), and Commitment (ethical view of the rights of others). Kohlberg and Kramer (1969) categorized the stages of moral development as Premoral (law and order); Morality of Conventional Role Conformity (avoiding disapproval of others); and Morality of Self-Accepted Moral Principles (avoiding self-condemnation) (Parrot, Cummings, & Marchell,

1994). By using these principles, facilitators will be better able to design programs that will be meaningful for the participants and to reach them on the emotional level.

Understanding and incorporating the life experiences of the participants also helps to make a program work. The more specific and local the program examples are, the more effective they will be. For example, if a member of a college (instead of a celebrity or someone from an institution 1,000 miles away) has been the victim of rape, the program participants are much more likely to believe that "it can and does happen here." Try to use statistics and examples from your community or college (such as mentioning the names of bars students frequent) to personalize the program for them.

## Employing Constructive Facilitation Skills

Special care needs to be taken in working with groups. It is important to have facilitators to whom the audience can relate. The trainers must be perceived as being there to help the participants avoid a problem rather than to point a finger at them. If the right kinds of insights don't come from the audience, they must be provided by the facilitator. If the facilitator has not been accepted by the group, his or her comments will fall on "deaf ears," or worse, on a hostile group.

## Retaining the Audience

Men at risk for sexual assault victimization and women who are potential assaulters may not view themselves as such. In addition, they are likely to think that only women are sexual assault victims and only men are assaulters. Therefore, if they are in a program in which the facilitator explains that this is a sexual assault prevention program to keep men from becoming victims and/or women from becoming victimizers, the facilitator may begin to lose the audience (literally if they leave, or, if it is a mandatory program, participants are likely to become hostile or to tune the facilitators out). Effective advertising and facilitation strategies will help avoid negative outcomes.

# ELEMENTS TO CONSIDER IN CREATING A SEXUAL ASSAULT PREVENTION PROGRAM

## Planning

### *Learn about the Group*

Talk with coaches, teachers, team captains, sorority/fraternity members or presidents, resident advisers, club advisors, or anyone else who can provide you with accurate information about the group you plan to address. Learn about their world. Use this information to tailor the program to make it specific to the participants.

### *Advertise*

If the program is not mandatory, the title must be intriguing enough to interest most of the target group. Therefore, titles such as "Men . . . Learn How to Avoid Being Sexually Assaulted" should not be used. Programs for potential male victims are likely to be most effective if the program is not directed at men exclusively and if all the examples are geared toward both men and women. Men are probably not going to come to a program that identifies them as potential targets, and women are not going to come if they are seen as potential victimizers. Therefore, the program should be advertised in a way to provide the information in the third person. For example, the title may be something like the following: "Help Prevent Someone You Care About from Being the Victim of a Sexual Assault." It may also be helpful to design a program for lesbian women and gay men and to market it as such to gay/lesbian groups.

### *Abusers or Victims May Be Present (So Should a Counselor)*

The facilitators must be aware that in any given group there may be both victims and assailants present. These participants may not identify themselves, but they are likely to become increasingly disturbed during the program (especially if victim-blaming comments are made). Therefore, it is best to have at least two facilitators, one leading the session, the other(s) observing the group for signs of someone who may appear to be upset. In that case, the person who is getting upset may be unobtrusively invited to step outside. A counselor or the facilitator (if she or he has counseling skills) may attempt to intervene and help the participant deal with his emotions. If not, an appropriate referral should be made sensitively.

### Content

*Statistics.* Facts need to be included, but they will not change attitudes, so use them sparingly. They tend just to bore people.

*Definitions.* Legal definitions of sexual assault for your jurisdiction are helpful.

*School Policies.* Students need to know what their rights and responsibilities are by virtue of being a student.

*Why Women and Men Feel and Think the Way They Do about Social Issues.* Peers, media, and family powerfully shape actions and beliefs. Programs need to address these influences, as well as people's fears, barriers to reporting, and gender issues.

*Listen to Your Instincts.* Before people are able to assert their needs and wants, they have to learn to listen to the messages their instincts give them regarding dangerous situations. They must learn that if something seems wrong, it probably is, and that they need to give themselves permission to get out of that situation. It is better for them to be embarrassed or to have made an incorrect assessment in the name of safety than to remain in a situation that gets out of control and in which one may become a victim.

## Types of Activities

### Engaging Techniques

Don't hesitate to use humor to engage the participants. They will be more open if the facilitator appears relaxed and genuine. Humor is a very helpful tool for disarming the audience, and although rape is not funny, the participants do need some way to discharge their tension, and laughter helps to do that. If the participants use graphic language, repeating it will disarm them and reduce the risk of them trying to make you "squirm." Ask them to define unfamiliar terms; this will show them that you are interested in what they have to say, and it will provide you with more information (Parrot, Cummings, & Marchell, 1994).

### Small-Group Discussions Guided by a Trained Facilitator

This technique is very important in allowing peer pressure to educate in a positive way. Even a group of hundreds of people can be broken up into small groups to discuss some important issues.

### Lecture

This is an effective technique to impart the factual information but should be used on a limited basis.

### Selected Activities

*Audiovisual Materials That Will Produce an Affective Response.* Because this is such a new and controversial area, it is nearly impossible to find any educational media developed for this audience. And because it will be very difficult for the participants to understand this issue, and to relate to the discussion, it is a helpful strategy to have some media to be used as a trigger or springboard. There are few good commercially produced educational videotapes that can be used in part as trigger films. Therefore, it is often more effective to use clips from entertainment movies available on video that the participants can relate to and that also depict male sexual assault victimization. A few films that may be useful for this purpose include, but are not limited to, *Disclosure* (forced sexual encounter of a male by a female acquaintance in a position of power), *Pulp Fiction* (male anal rape by a male stranger), *Fatal Attraction* (coerced male sex by a female acquaintance), *The Prince of Tides* (childhood anal rape by a male stranger), and *Deliverance* (male anal rape by a male stranger).

*Assertiveness Training.* Because sexual assault sometimes occurs when people are not able to make their wishes understood or heard, an activity on assertiveness is an important element to include in a program to prevent sexual assault victimization. "Assertiveness in Our Lives" (see Appendix A) encourages communication about sex and will allow the facilitator to make some assessments about the group. For example, as a result of doing this activity with a group, the facilitator will be able to make an assessment of the group regarding their willingness to participate openly and honestly, whether they are liberal or conservative (Parrot, 1990) .

There are several other activities that can be done with groups to deal with the issues of sexual assertiveness skills of the participants (see Appendices B, C, and D). The "Sexual Assertiveness Questionnaire" (Appendix B) is designed for nonassertive groups that are not initially willing to share information with others. Once members of the group have completed the questionnaire independently, they should be asked to share their comments with others in a discussion format (Parrot, 1990).

The "Sexual Assertiveness Continuum" (Appendix C) can be used in place of the previous activity. Participants can complete this individually, or, as a large-group activity, they can place their bodies on a line on the floor that corresponds to the continuum values (1–5) for a specific question. Then they are stating their opinions, albeit nonverbally. They should be invited to explain why they are where they are on the line; a discussion usually ensues (Parrot, 1991). "Sexual Assertiveness Using 'I' Statements" (Appendix D) is probably best as a homework assignment for partners in a relationship to complete in a private setting (Parrot, 1991).

## Reporting

Male victims of sexual assault need to understand that being forced to have sex is illegal, and that they have a right to report the crime. Unfortunately, there is a widely held perception that male victims enjoyed the assault and are more responsible for their own assault than are female victims. Therefore, male victims are less likely to report the assault to the police or other authorities. But even if they choose not to report the assault to authorities, they should be encouraged to seek counseling to deal with their feelings as a result of the assault.

## Counseling

Male victims of sexual assault often experience rape trauma syndrome (Sarrel & Masters, 1982), as well as isolation, because they fear that no one will believe them, understand them, or support them (Smith, Pine, & Hawley, 1988). Women and men who are sexually assaultive are more likely to have experienced childhood sexual abuse (Anderson, 1996; Rivera & Widom, 1990). Therefore, both victims and perpetrators should be encouraged to find a supportive therapist who has training in sexual victimization to help them deal with their dysfunctional feelings.

## Closure

Participants need strategies for prevention that they can actually use. These are best if they come from the participants themselves. In addition, they need to know what to do if they encounter a friend who has been sexually assaulted, who is considering committing a sexual assault, or who already has. Counseling center and police numbers are important to provide, as well as pamphlets that provide information on the points mentioned in this paragraph.

## CONCLUSION

A good rape prevention program should empower students to challenge and refute behaviors such as aggression, sexism, peer harassment, and alcohol and other drug abuse that can contribute to the likelihood of sexual assault. Participants should also feel that they have learned new strategies to resist peer pressure and avoid involvement in sexual assault. We must be careful to avoid programs that simply tell participants to change their behavior without telling them how they should behave. We will not be effective in changing attitudes if we do not reach the participants on the affective (feeling) level. Participants have to not only understand the dysfunction of rape culturally but they also need to empathize with the pain of sexual assault.

## APPENDIX A. Assertiveness in Our Lives

(Time necessary depends on group size; 10 to 30 minutes)

### Introduction

Introduce the session by using a nonthreatening example that relates to assertiveness but does not reduce discomfort associated with a discussion of sexuality. This is an example that relates to smoking in an elevator. Tell participants the following:

- Imagine you are all nonsmokers who hate cigarette smoke.
- You are waiting for an elevator on the first floor, and you must ride to the third floor.
- When it arrives, you get on it, and so does someone with a lit cigarette.
- What do you do? (Try to elicit as many different responses as possible.)
- Would your response be different if there were a "No Smoking" sign in the elevator?
- Would your response be different if this person were your supervisor or teacher?

### Processing

The responses probably ranged from very nonassertive (such as "I would hold my breath," or "I would get off the elevator and walk"), to aggressive (such as "Cigarettes are disgusting," or "I would put it out for him or her"), to lying (such as "I am allergic to cigarette smoke"). Did the types of responses differ by sex? If so, why?

Most likely, very few answers were assertive, and most would not fit into the formula of "When you do *x*, I feel *y*, and I want you to do *z*." Assertions are difficult with people we do not know but may even be more difficult with people we do know.

There are several reasons why it is even more difficult to be assertive in a sexual interaction:

1. You must put your desires over those of someone you care about when you are asserting for something contrary to the desires of others.

*Note.* From Parrot (1991, pp. 129–130). Copyright 1991 by Learning Publications. Reprinted by permission.

2. You are not usually taught or encouraged to talk about sex or use sexual words in normal conversation.

3. Communication about sex often takes place in the context of "game playing," not honest communication about feelings.

4. We are not generally expected to share our feelings with others, especially if that sharing may make us vulnerable.

5. We may not be absolutely sure about what we want sexually.

6. We have been receiving conflicting messages from many different sources in our lives about what is correct and how we should behave sexually.

7. We can use the law or our health as reasons to be assertive about smoking because smoking, may be hazardous to health and is illegal in some nonventilated public areas. It is not always illegal or unhealthy to engage in behaviors such as "petting."

8. Either men or women are allowed to dislike smoking, but neither sex is supposed to dislike sex, and each sex is bound by certain restrictive sex roles.

## APPENDIX B. Sexual Assertiveness Questionnaire

Directions: Check which category best indicates your response to the questions below.

|  | Almost always | Sometimes | Almost never |
|---|---|---|---|
| How often would/do you . . . | | | |
| 1. Make your own decision regarding intercourse or other sexual activity regardless of your partner's wishes? | _____ | _____ | _____ |
| 2. Use or not use birth control regardless of your partner's wishes? | _____ | _____ | _____ |
| 3. Tell your partner when you want to make love? | _____ | _____ | _____ |
| 4. Tell your partner when you don't want to make love? | _____ | _____ | _____ |
| 5. Tell your partner you won't have intercourse without birth control? | _____ | _____ | _____ |
| 6. Tell your partner you want to make love different? | _____ | _____ | _____ |

*Note.* From Parrot (1991, pp. 137–138). Copyright 1991 by Learning Publications. Reprinted by permission.

7. Masturbate to orgasm? _____ _____ _____
8. Tell your partner s/he is being too rough? _____ _____ _____
9. Tell your partner you want to be hugged or cuddled without sex? _____ _____ _____
10. Tell a relative you're uncomfortable being hugged or kissed in certain ways? _____ _____ _____
11. Ask your partner if s/he has been examined for sexually transmitted diseases? _____ _____ _____

## APPENDIX C. Sexual Assertiveness Continuum

Directions: Circle the number on the continuum to indicate the strength of your agreement with the statement on either end of the continuum.

1. In a sexual relationship, if something, bothers you, you should always tell your partner.

   In a sexual relationship, it is better not to tell your partner if something is bothering you.

   1        2        3            4        5

2. When having sex with a new person, it is best to state what you want and don't want before you actually do anything sexual.

   When having sex with a new person it is best to allow the relationship to develop and to try to nonverbally alter your partner's behaviors that you don't like.

   1        2        3            4        5

3. When would you bring up the possibility of having a sexually transmitted disease with a partner? (Check one.)
   _____ When making the date
   _____ Before taking clothes off
   _____ Before sex
   _____ After first sexual act
   _____ After one of you has been told you have an STD
   _____ Never

*Note.* From Parrot (1991, p. 139). Copyright 1991 by Learning Publications. Reprinted by permission.

4. "No" means NO.              "No" means maybe or yes.

   1          2          3          4          5


## APPENDIX D.  Sexual Assertiveness Using "I" Statements

### Introduction

There are probably many things you like about your partner interpersonally and sexually. There are also some things you would like to change. If you don't have a partner right now, you still probably have an idea of what you would like and dislike in an interpersonal and sexual relationship.

A very difficult communication task is to let your partner know what you don't like in a way that will not cause hard feelings or anger. One way to do this is to explain that you don't like the act but you like the person and you like many other acts performed by your partner. In addition, if you can suggest what you would like instead, your partner may not feel helpless when you say what you don't like.

It is easier to hear criticism when:

- Positive feedback is given at the same time.
- The act, not the person is rejected.
- The criticism does not come at a time of "high emotional investment" (e.g., tell your partner at breakfast rather than when you are making love).
- Only one criticism is given in a sitting, so the person doesn't feel like there is nothing he or she can do right.
- The message is clear, and the verbal message matches the nonverbal message.

### Directions

*For short-term relationships (if this is your first sexual interaction with this partner):*

If you feel you can't tell your partner what you like and don't like before you begin to interact sexually, then tell him or her immediately when a behavior you don't like begins.

1. Use the formula "When you do x, I feel y and I want you to do z."
2. Be consistent with your verbal and nonverbal messages.

*Note.* From Parrot (1991, pp. 145–147). Copyright 1991 by Learning Publications. Reprinted by permission.

3. Reject the behavior, not the person (e.g., don't say, "You are a terrible lover," or "Can't you do anything right?" but: "When you kiss my neck in that way, I feel uncomfortable and I'd like you to stop kissing my neck.") Make sure the feeling you indicate is clearly negative.

4. Do not allow the behavior to continue once you have clearly stated your displeasure with it.

5. If your partner does not stop that behavior, ask him or her to explain what they think you said. If your partner doesn't understand, explain again using different words, and check to make sure your verbal and nonverbal messages are consistent. If he or she understands, but still will not stop, GET OUT OF THE SITUATION; your wishes are being ignored.

*For long-term relationships:*

*To be done in the session:* Make a list of the things you like and dislike about what your partner does sexually. Now circle those things in the "dislike" column that you really want changed and leave the items that you could live with. Now number the circled items in the order of most important to least important ("I" being the most important).

*To be done at home with your partner:* When you talk with your partner about this, have him or her make a list for you too. Then set aside a time when you will not be interrupted to discuss these issues. Tell your partner one thing from your "like" list, then one from your "dislike" list, and then finally another from your "like" list. When you are discussing the item from the "dislike" list, be specific, provide an alternate or substitute behavior, and put the "dislike" item in the formula, "When you do $x$, I feel $y$." For example: "When you ask me to give you a massage, but you won't give me one afterwards, I feel exploited or unimportant, I wouldn't feel that way if you would give me a back massage too." Then ask your partner to repeat back to you the positives, the negatives, the feelings you stated, and the suggestions you made. Once your partner has clearly heard all of what you have said, then switch roles, and your partner will tell you what he or she does not like.

Work on only one item at a time, and when you have mastered that, then go on to another one on your "dislike" list. Continue to revise your lists, and keep moving the improved behaviors over to your "like" side. This process could take months, but the results will be worth it.

# REFERENCES

Aizenman, M., & Kelley, G. (1988). The incidence of violence and acquaintance rape in dating relationships among college men and women. *Journal of College Student Development, 29,* 305–311.

Allgeier, E., & McCormick, N. (Eds.). (1983). *Changing boundaries: Gender roles and sexual behavior.* Palo Alto, CA: Mayfield.

Anderson, P. (1996). Correlates of college women's self-reports of heterosexual aggression. *Sexual Abuse: A Journal of Research and Treatment, 8*(2), 121–131.

Brehm, S. (1985). *Intimate relationships.* New York: Random House.

Clark, R., & Hatfield, E. (1989). Gender differences in receptivity to sexual offers. *Journal of Psychology and Human Sexuality, 2,* 39–55.

Doyle, J. (1983). *The male experience.* Dubuque, IA: William C. Brown.

Goyer, P., & Eddleman, H. (1984). Same-sex rape of nonincarcerated men. *American Journal of Psychiatry, 141,* 576–579.

Groth, A. N., & Burgess, A. W. (1980). Male rape: Offenders and victims. *American Journal of Psychiatry, 137,* 806–810.

Hickson, R., Davies, P., Hunt, A., Weatherburn, P., McManis, T., & Coxon, A. (1994). Gay men as victims of nonconsensual sex. *Archives of Sexual Behavior, 23*(3), 281–294.

Kaufman, A., Divasto, P., Jackson, R., Voorhees, D., & Christy, J. (1980). Male rape victims: Noninstitutionalized assault. *American Journal of Psychiatry, 137,* 221–223.

Kohlberg, L., & Kramer, R. (1969). Continuities and discontinuities in childhood and adult development. *Human Development, 12,* 93–120.

Komarovsky, M. (1976). *Dilemmas of masculinity: A study of college youth.* New York: Norton.

Muehlenhard, C., & Cook, S. (1988). Men's self-reports of unwanted sexual activity. *Journal of Sex Research, 24,* 58–72.

Myers, M. (1989). Men sexually assaulted as adults and sexually abused as boys. *Archives of Sexual Behavior, 18,* 203–215.

O'Sullivan, L., & Byers, E. (1993). Eroding stereotypes: College women's attempts to influence reluctant male sexual partners. *Journal of Sex Research, 30,* 270–282.

Parrot, A. (1991). *Acquaintance rape and sexual assault prevention training manual* (5th ed.). Holmes Beach, FL: Learning Publications.

Parrot, A., Cummings, N., & Marchell, T. (1994). *Rape 101: Sexual assault prevention for college athletes.* Holmes Beach, FL: Learning Publications.

Parrot, A., Cummings, N., Marchell, T., & Hofher, J. (1994). A rape awareness and prevention model for male athletes. *Journal of American College Health, 42,* 179–184.

Perry, W. (1970). *Forms of intellectual and ethical development in the college years.* New York: Holt, Rinehart & Winston.

Rivera, B., & Widom, C. (1990). Childhood victimization and violent offending. *Violence and Victims, 5*(1), 19–35.

Rosenfeld, A. (1982, September). When women rape men. *Omni,* pp. 28, 194.

Sanday, P. (1990). *Fraternity gang rape.* New York: New York University Press.

Sarrel, P., & Masters, W. (1982). Sexual molestation of men by women. *Archives of Sexual Behavior, 11,* 117–131.

Smith, R., Pine, C., & Hawley, M. (1988). Social cognitions about adult male victims of female sexual assault. *Journal of Sex Research, 24,* 101–112.

Struckman-Johnson, C. (1991). Male victims of acquaintance rape. In A. Parrot & L. Bechhofer (Eds.), *Acquaintance rape: The hidden crime* (pp. 192–214). New York: Wiley.

Waterman, C., Dawson, L., & Bologna, M. (1989). Sexual coercion in gay male and lesbian relationships: Predictors and implications for support services. *Journal of Sex Research, 26,* 118–124.

Weis, K., & Borges, S. (1973). Victimology and rape: The case of the legitimate victim. *Issues in Criminology, 8,* 71–115.

Zilbergeld, B. (1978). *Male sexuality: A guide to sexual fulfillment.* New York: Bantam.

## RECOMMENDED RESOURCES

Beneke, T. (1983). *Men on rape.* New York: St. Martin's Press.

Coronet/MI Film and Video (Producers). *Can a guy say no?* [Video]. (Available from the producers at 108 Willmont Road, Deerfield, IL 60015; 1-800-621-2131)

Farrell, W. (1988). *Why men are the way they are.* New York: Berkley Books.

# Postscript:
# Where Do We Go
# from Here?

PETER B. ANDERSON
CINDY STRUCKMAN-JOHNSON

As discussed in Section I of this volume, there are many research and conceptual issues that have yet to be addressed in the area of women's sexual aggression. We conclude this volume with our personal perspectives and recommendations for future research. It is evident that this is a highly controversial area and that the definitions selected by researchers will most likely reflect their theoretical perspectives, personal values, and the political climate of the times. We recognize that portraying women as potentially sexually harmful is an unpopular concept, particularly in light of the decades it has taken for researchers to demonstrate the sobering problems of male sexual assault of women. However, social science should not be driven by popularity or suitability of topics but by the need to understand behavior in all of its variations.

## DEFINITIONS OF SEXUAL AGGRESSION

Presently, it is difficult to assess the prevalence of sexual aggression among female or male populations because of the diversity of terms and definitions in use. The original definition of "rape" as a crime, derived from British common law, was "carnal knowledge of a woman by force and against her will" (Largen, 1988). As discussed by Allgeier and Lamping in Chapter 3, feminism and social concerns have led to some changes in the legal definitions and terms related to rape. For example, a "state of incapacity" to give consent (e.g., unconsciousness; purposefully giving someone alcohol or drugs with the intent to diminish their capacity) is grounds for a rape charge in many states. There is also a trend to expand the limitation of vaginal–penile intercourse to include any sexual penetration, oral sex, and genital touching in legal definitions of rape. Many states have implemented gender-neutral terms to protect male receivers of sexual aggression. And the term "sexual assault" is used in conjunction with the term "rape" in many statutes (Largen, 1988; Searles & Berger, 1987).

The social pressures that have brought about legal reforms have also influenced social scientists' definitions of rape and sexual aggression (Muehlenhard, Harney, & Jones, 1992). In research, the concept of sexual aggression has been broadened to include a range of sexual activities (e.g., kissing, touching, sexual penetration) enacted by a variety of nonforceful and forceful tactics. However, there are inconsistencies in how researchers employ specific definitions and terms. Some researchers may distinguish "rape" behaviors that meet legal definitions of rape from less serious acts of sexual aggression (e.g., Koss, Gidycz, & Wisniewski, 1987; Russell, 1984). Others may use the term "sexual assault" to refer to *all* sexually aggressive behaviors, including attempts at sexual touching brought about by nonforceful tactics (e.g., George, Winfield, & Blazer, 1992; Sorenson, Stein, Siegel, Golding, & Burnam, 1987). These differences in the use of terms help explain the widely divergent rates of sexual aggression reported in the literature.

In the past we have used different definitions of sexual aggression in our own research and have struggled with the meaning and appropriateness of terms. Nevertheless, as a starting point, we propose that "sexual aggression" and "sexual coercion" be used as *general* terms encompassing the full range of behaviors that are employed by adults to obtain unwanted sexual contact with adults or adolescents. One definition of sexual aggression that we favor is "the use of pressure or force to obtain sexual contact with another person against their will" (Sorenson, et al., 1987). Pressure tactics would include a wide variety of actions such as persistent sexual stimulation, persistent arguments, deception, emotional manipulation, threats of self-harm, blackmail, and inappropriate use of one's authority (e.g., employer, teacher, religious leader). Force tactics would include physical restraint, intimidation by physical size or power, threats of physical harm, actual physical harm, and the use of a weapon to threaten or harm.

The categorization of tactics involving alcohol and drugs is difficult and requires careful discernment. Sometimes people have mutually consenting sexual contact when one or both parties drink or take drugs to the extent that the ability to give consent is compromised. We suggest that the incident be considered a pressure tactic if one person uses the other's voluntary intoxication to obtain unwanted sexual contact. When the situation involves one person giving alcohol or drugs to another with the intent to diminish their capacity to give consent, the incident would be categorized as a force tactic.

When reporting adult sexual aggression estimates, we recommend that researchers distinguish between rates for pressured and for forced incidents and present statistics for the different types of strategies used. The reader is then in a position to judge the severity of incidents and to draw comparisons to estimates reported in other studies. Finally, the term "sexual abuse" would best remain separately applied to sexual aggression involving children, as it is often used now.

## ASSESSMENT OF SEXUAL AGGRESSION

We believe that there is a need to improve how sexual aggression is measured in present day research. It is our opinion that in many studies, too much is inferred from too little information. We agree with contributing authors Allgeier and Lamping (Chapter 3) that researchers should be cautious with simple assessment techniques whereby respondents answer "yes" or "no" questions about perpetrating or receiving sexual aggression. The respondents and the researchers may have different interpretations of the meaning of these items. Thus, for future research, we recommend collecting descriptive information to aid in classifying sexually aggressive events.

Dual assessment of female and male sexual aggression will require modification of sexual aggression questionnaires traditionally designed to measure female victimization. Some researchers have reworded the Sexual Experiences Survey (SES; Koss & Oros, 1982) so that both men and women can answer questions about committing and receiving sexually coercive acts (e.g., Anderson & Aymami, 1993; LaVoie & Poitras, 1996). Researchers who develop their own measures of sexual aggression should avoid the use of terms that may have different meanings for women and men. For example, if one asks, "Have you ever been sexually aggressive with a dating partner?" women may think that the question refers to making direct sexual offers, whereas a man may think the question refers to the use of physical force. We recommend using more specific questions. An example would be, "Have you ever pressured or forced a man/woman to have sexual contact against their will?" with follow-up questions that determine what type of pressure or force strategy was used.

We recommend that researchers collect at least four types of data about sexual interactions under investigation: (1) the specific behaviors used to accomplish sexual contact (e.g., pressure tactics, force tactics); (2) sexual outcome (e.g., touching vs. intercourse); (3) evidence for the receiver's lack of consent; and (4) context of the situation (e.g., relationship of couple, events leading up to the incident). With this level of descriptive detail, one could develop a reasonable strategy for categorizing the sexually coercive behavior of *individuals,* regardless of their gender.

As discussed above, the practice of reporting general sexual aggression or sexual assault estimates without qualifying the types of incidents included makes it difficult to discern the severity level of cases. In our opinion, an incident between an adult man and woman involving physically forced intercourse is more serious than an incident involving genital touching brought about by verbal pressure.

## Sexual Outcome

Every sexual aggression survey should be able to measure for "sexual outcome" to determine if the incident involved touching or more intimate varieties of intercourse. For dual assessment of female and male sexual aggression, the measures should include a range of sexual activities that can happen to both sexes. Examples could include categories for "fondling her breasts," "fondling his penis/testicles," "oral sex" and "fellatio" (a very common act perpetrated by sexually aggressive women), and "anal penetration," because sexually aggressive women and men sometimes commit sodomy using objects or fingers.

## Lack of Consent

Establishing lack of consent is integral to our definition of sexual aggression, but, again, care must be taken in measurement. For example, it could be misleading to focus only on verbal messages (i.e., "did you say 'no' to sex") in asking questions about consent. Research has established that both men and women engage in token denials—saying "no" when they really mean "yes"—and token consent—saying "yes" when sex is not wanted (Sprecher, Hatfield, Cortese, Potapova, & Levitskaya, 1994). There are also situations in which couples engage in rituals of "mock force" or consensual sadomasochistic behaviors during which men and women say "no" as part of a role play of force and submission. One way to assess consent is to ask clearly and directly. Consent is often assessed in surveys by asking respondents if sexual contact occurred "when 'the person' (either you, if you are the receiver, or someone else, if you are the initiator) did not want to have sex." However, like Allgeier and Lamping (Chapter 3, this volume), we believe that instead of asking if sex occurred "when the person did not want to have sex," it may be preferable to ask if sexual contact happened "against someone's will." Researchers can also ask respondents to explain in their own words if and how consent was given or denied.

## Context

Here we offer the recommendation of Byers and O'Sullivan (see Chapter 8, this volume) to collect information about the *context* of the situation, such as setting, the relationship between the persons, the events that led up to the incident, and the emotional impact of the event upon the receiver. The meaning and value of any sexual encounter is best defined by the actors involved and with the contextual framework of the encounter taken into account. The macro- and micromessages that women and men receive through their individual life circumstances, based on their regional, economic, familial, ethnic, spiritual, and educational circumstances and their peer group norms, are critical determinants of definitions of their behaviors. These data also help clarify strategies and consent status for researchers. For example, we have had respondents check categories such as "used physical force" or "got you drunk," which would be classified as sexual assault or rape. However, the respondents' written descriptions revealed that the force was actually part of a sex game or that the intoxication was voluntary and mutual. Thus, contextual information may greatly improve the accuracy of categorizing sexually aggressive events.

## IDEAS FOR FUTURE RESEARCH
## ON SEXUALLY AGGRESSIVE WOMEN

We believe there is exciting work to be done on explanations for why women pressure or force men to have sex. Depending on one's theoretical framework, a variety of hypotheses can be generated. Below we list some of the more promising proposals derived from the literature and our own ideas.

### Social Learning Perspectives

Adversarial beliefs about relationships and the acceptance of sexual stereotypes about men have all been linked to women's sexual aggression (Anderson 1996 and Chapter 4, this volume; Clements-Schreiber & Rempel, 1995). Anderson (1996) has presented evidence that women who hold adversarial beliefs about relationships are somewhat more likely than other women to use sexually coercive tactics with men. Adversarial beliefs in sum are: "the belief that relationships are fundamentally exploitative, that each party to them is manipulative, sly, cheating, opaque to the other's understanding, and not to be trusted" (Burt, 1980, p. 218). Similarly, women who accept stereotypes that men are "always sexually ready" and "easily controlled by the sexual manipulations of women" may actually perceive their actions as positive because they think that men want them to behave in an aggressive manner (Clements-Schreiber & Rempel, 1995). This could be one reason why, in prior research on women's and men's self-reports of women's sexual aggression, women report giving less aggression than men report receiving (Anderson & Aymami, 1993). Currently, Canadian researchers Clements-Schreiber and Rempel are developing a survey to measure an array of negative male sexual stereotypes. Once completed, this measure could be used in a variety of ways to assess the beliefs systems of coercive and noncoercive women.

Women also learn about sexual behavior through school curricula at all levels and from the media. Is sex education one of the mediating factors in sexual aggression? Lottes and Weinberg (1996) raised this question when they published a report showing that young American women and men exhibit significantly higher levels of sexual aggression than their counterparts in Sweden. These authors suggest that the Swedish policy of teaching "relationship ethics" to schoolchildren may decrease sexual aggression in dating situations. One research idea would be to expand Burt's (1980) work on relationship beliefs and measure the impact of women's relationship "ethics" on their sexually aggressive behaviors.

Women most likely learn more about sexual behavior from the media than they do in sex education classes. To what extent have the pervasive and sometimes explicit sexual themes in advertising, movies, popular prime-time shows, daytime talk shows, and women's magazines influenced the sexual aggressiveness of young women?

## Personality and Trait Approach

Dr. William Prendergast (1979) developed a theory about rapists based on his work in prisons with incarcerated male offenders. He believes that sexual violence is the result of an inadequate personality formation combined with childhood trauma. Other more recent research has linked the experience of childhood sexual abuse with men who are sexual offenders (Haapasalo & Kankkonen, 1997). Anderson (Chapter 4, this volume) has demonstrated a relationship between a woman's experience of past sexual abuse and her likelihood of using sexually aggressive tactics to attempt sexual contact with adult or adolescent men. Shea (Chapter 5, this volume) has evidence that college women who use verbal coercion to obtain sex share common traits, including a tendency to be power-oriented and sexually motivated and to view relationships as a means for gaining advantages.

Research by Struckman-Johnson and Struckman-Johnson (Chapter 7, this volume) suggest that the sexually coercive behavior of women may be motivated by a misguided desire for intimacy. In their surveys, many men say that they have been sexually exploited by "unsuitable" or unattractive women who had crushes on them and took advantage of the men's state of intoxication to have sex. Thus, the desire to start a relationship with an attractive, but "unattainable," man may lead some women to use sexual aggression. Motives could be assessed by asking women to cite and explain their reasons for pressuring or forcing men to have sex.

In future research, it would be interesting to determine if there exists a "prototype" or array of personality characteristics of the sexually coercive woman. Potential predictive traits may be related to extroversion, impulsiveness, emotional stability, sociosexual orientation (Simpson & Gangestad, 1991), and self- or sexual self-esteem.

## Evolutionary and Sociobiological Theories

According to sociobiological theories, men make sexual initiatives to multiple partners in order to insure that their genes survive. Women, on the other hand, restrict making sexual overtures because they must select an appropriate man who has the resources to provide for her and her children (Haas & Haas, 1993). However, Buss and Schmidt (1993) have suggested that women also have "short term" mating strategies that are motivated by spontaneous sexual attraction to a particular man, even though the interaction has low relationship potential.

Ellis has proposed that sexually coercive women may have higher levels of male sex hormones, which are manifested in a higher sex drive and/or a willingness to use physically forceful tactics (Chapter 6, this volume). Previous researchers (Dabbs, Ruback, Frady, Hopper, & Sgoutas, 1988) have investigated the relationship between testosterone levels and criminal behavior among women.

Ellis's proposal could be investigated by expanding the work of Dabbs et al. by using saliva tests to assess the testosterone levels of sexually aggressive and nonaggressive women. Another approach would be to test the relationship between the use of sexually coercive behaviors by women and their time of ovulation, when sexual interest is known to peak (Van Goozen, Wiegant, Endert, Helmond, & Van de Poll, 1997).

## Alcohol

Previous studies have suggested that women engage in coercive sexual behavior when they or their male target or both have been drinking (Muehlenhard & Cook, 1988; Struckman-Johnson & Struckman-Johnson, 1994). Are advertising campaigns linking alcohol to fun and sex influencing women to be sexually aggressive? Are women (like men) using alcohol as an excuse for their sexually aggressive behavior? It would be interesting in future research to ask both female sexual aggressors and male receivers to estimate the causal role of alcohol in the incident.

## CONCLUSION

Throughout this volume we have discussed the multitude of problems that have influenced research on sexually aggressive women. They include social prejudice against an unpopular topic, double standards and inconsistencies in definitions, and deficiencies in measurement. Still, we remain optimistic and excited about this area of research. We know that the promising questions that we have posed for future research are but a few of the unlimited possibilities. Other psychological theories, such as individual readiness, cognitive processing, moral development, and reward theory, could all provide plausible and testable hypotheses related to women's sexual aggression. By approaching research in this area from as many perspectives as possible, knowledge of this phenomenon will be rapidly advanced.

In closing, we hope that the challenges presented by the information and ideas in this book will allow us to understand and define sexual aggression in new ways. We trust that this book will stimulate more research on the dynamics of sexual interactions, the initiation of programs to help people heal from sexual trauma when it occurs, and more beneficial, mutually consenting sexual interactions.

## REFERENCES

Anderson, P. (1996). Correlates of college women's self-reports of hetero-sexual aggression. *Sexual Abuse: A Journal of Research and Treatment,* 8(2), 121–131.

Anderson, P., & Aymami, R. (1993). Reports of female initiation of sexual contact: Male and female differences. *Archives of Sexual Behavior, 22*(4), 335–343.

Burt, M. (1980). Cultural myths and supports for rape. *Journal or Person-ality and Social Psychology, 38*(2), 217–230.

Buss, D. M., & Schmidt, D. P. (1993). Sexual strategies theory: An evolutionary perspective on human mating. *Psychological Review, 100,* 202–232.

Clements-Schreiber, M. E., & Rempel, J. K. (1995, October). *Women's acceptance of male sexual stereotypes: Does "no" mean "keep trying"?* Paper presented at the 22nd annual meeting of the Canadian Sex Research Forum, Banff, Alberta, Canada.

Dabbs, J. M., Ruback, B. R., Frady, R. L., Hopper, C. H., & Sgoutas, D. S. (1988). Sliva testosterone and criminal violence among women. *Personality and Individual Differences, 9,* 269–275.

George, L., Winfield, I., & Blazer, D. (1992). Sociocultural factors in sexual assault: Comparison of two representative samples of women. *Journal of Social Issues, 48,* 105–125.

Haapasalo, J., & Kankkonen, O. (1997). Self-reported childhood abuse among sex and violent offenders. *Archives of Sexual Behavior, 26,* 421–432.

Haas, K., & Haas, A. (1993). *Understanding sexuality* (3rd ed.). Boston: Mosby.

Koss, M., Gidycz, C., & Wisniewski, N. (1987). The scope of rape: Incidence and prevalence of sexual aggression and victimization in a national sample of higher education students. *Journal of Consulting and Clinical Psychology, 55,* 162–170.

Koss, M. P., & Oros, C. J. (1982). Sexual Experiences Survey: A research instrument investigating sexual aggression and victimization. *Journal of Consulting and Clinical Psychology, 50,* 455–457.

Largen, M. A. (1988). Rape-law reform: An analysis. In A. W. Burgess (Ed.), *Rape and sexual assault II* (pp. 271–292). New York: Garland.

Lavoie, F., & Poitras, M. (1996). A study of the prevalence of sexual coercion in adolescent dating relationships in a Quebec sample. *Victims and Violence, 10,* 125–139.

Lottes, I., & Weinberg, M. (1996). Sexual coercion among university students: A comparison of the United States and Sweden. *Journal of Sex Research, 34,* 67–76.

Muehlenhard, C., & Cook, S. (1988). Men's self-reports of unwanted sexual activity. *Journal of Sex Research, 24,* 58–72.

Muehlenhard, C., Harney, P., & Jones, J. (1992). From "victim precipitated rape" to "date rape": How far have we come? *Annual Review of Sex Research, 3,* 219–252.

Prendergast, W. (1979). The sex offender: How to spot him before it's too late. *Sexology, 46*(2), 46–51.

Russell, D. E. H. (1984). *Sexual exploitation: Rape, child sexual abuse, and workplace harassment.* Beverly Hills, CA: Sage.

Searles, P., & Berger, R. (1987). The current status of rape reform legislation: An examination of state statutes. *Women's Rights Law Reporter, 10,* 25–43.

Simpson, J. A., & Gangestad, S. W. (1991). Individual differences in sociosexuality: Evidence for convergent and discriminant validity. *Journal of Personality and Social Psychology, 60,* 870-883.

Sorenson, S., Stein, J., Siegel, J., Golding, J., & Burnam, M. (1987). The prevalence of adult sexual assault: The Los Angeles Epidemiologic Catchment Area Project. *American Journal of Epidemiology, 126,* 1154–1164.

Sprecher, S., Hatfield, E., Cortese, A., Potapova, E., & Levitskaya, A. (1994). Token resistance to sexual intercourse and consent to unwanted sexual intercourse: College students' dating experiences in three countries. *Journal of Sex Research, 31,* 125–132.

Struckman-Johnson, C., & Struckman-Johnson, D. (1994). Men pressured and forced into sexual experience. *Archives of Sexual Behavior, 23,* 93–114.

Van Goozen, S., Wiegant, V., Endert, E., Helmond, F., & Van de Poll, N. (1997). Psychoendocrinological assessment of the menstrual cycle: The relationship between hormones, sexuality, and mood. *Archives of Sexual Behavior, 26*(4), 359–382.

# Index